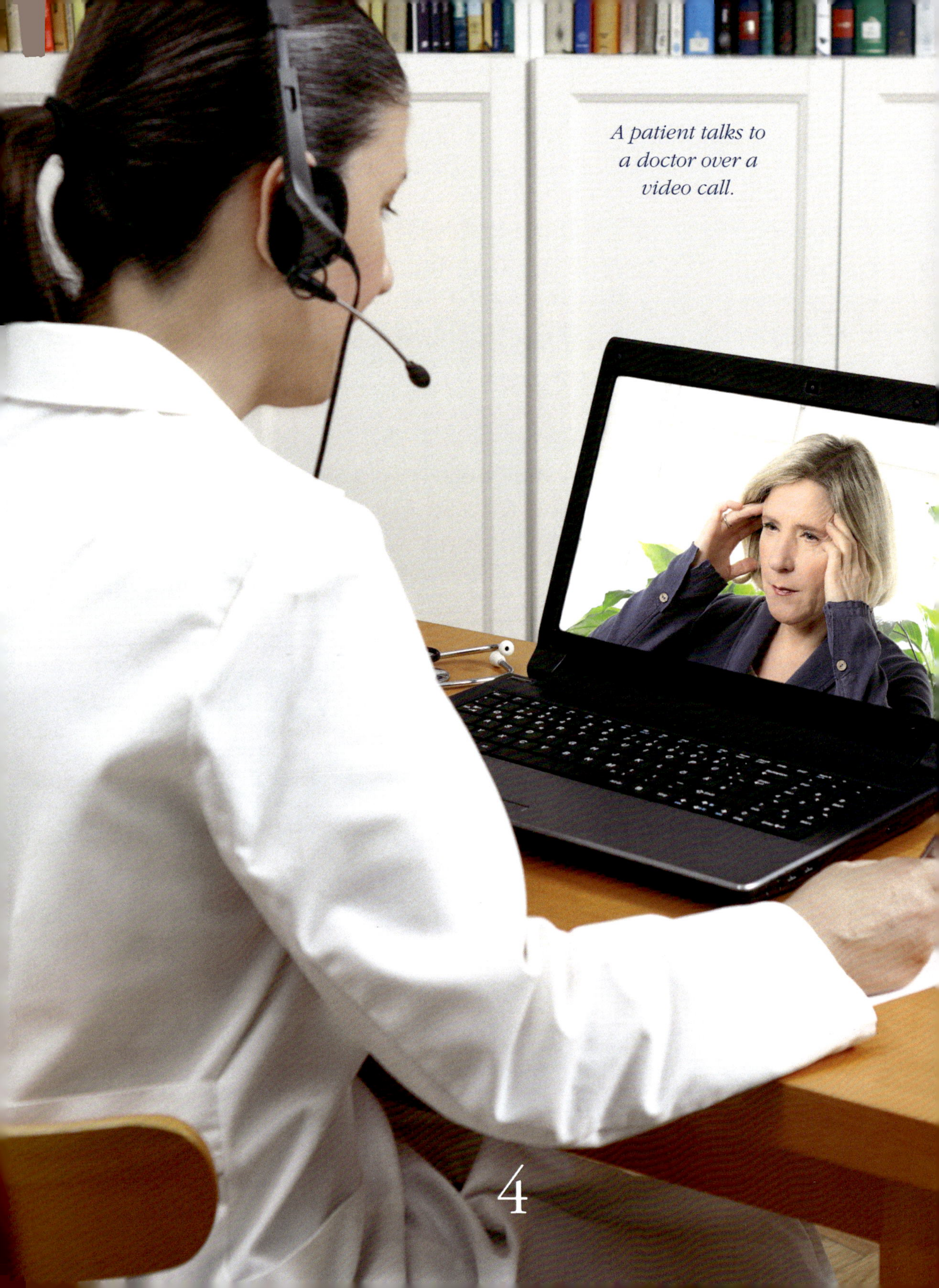

A patient talks to a doctor over a video call.

AI IN THE WORLD

12 USES FOR ARTIFICIAL INTELLIGENCE IN HEALTHCARE

Table of Contents

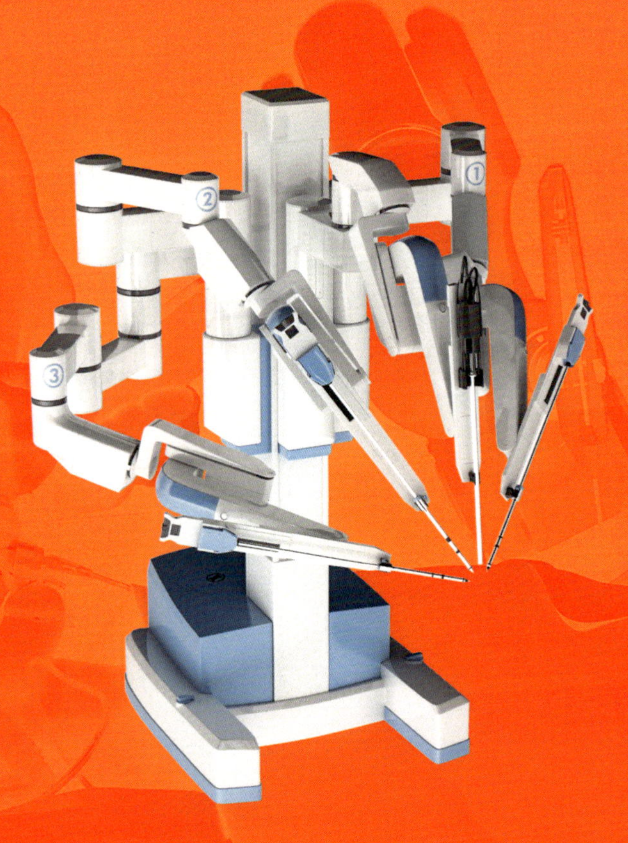

AI Helps Doctors Take *Better Notes*

1

An American visits the doctor around three times a year. At each visit, important information is taken. Doctors and nurses make notes. These go into a system. Other healthcare people can find it. They help track a person's health. A doctor may find a pattern of symptoms. But sometimes, they miss patterns. Artificial intelligence (AI) can help with this.

Ambience is an AI tool. It works on laptops and phones. It records all appointments. It takes notes on what tests were done. The doctor looks at them and gives their approval. Then Ambience sends summaries to patients. Their families and their caregivers also get copies. This makes sure everyone has the same information. Ambience AI can write in different languages too.

Insurance companies also use this tool. They need to know what procedures were done. Ambience breaks it down. Each visit is documented. The tool helps the insurance provider decide how much the visit costs.

Patients may change doctors. Or they need to see a **specialist**. Ambience helps in this as well. It writes letters to explain the person's medical history. The new doctor can see what has been tried before. Less time is wasted between care.

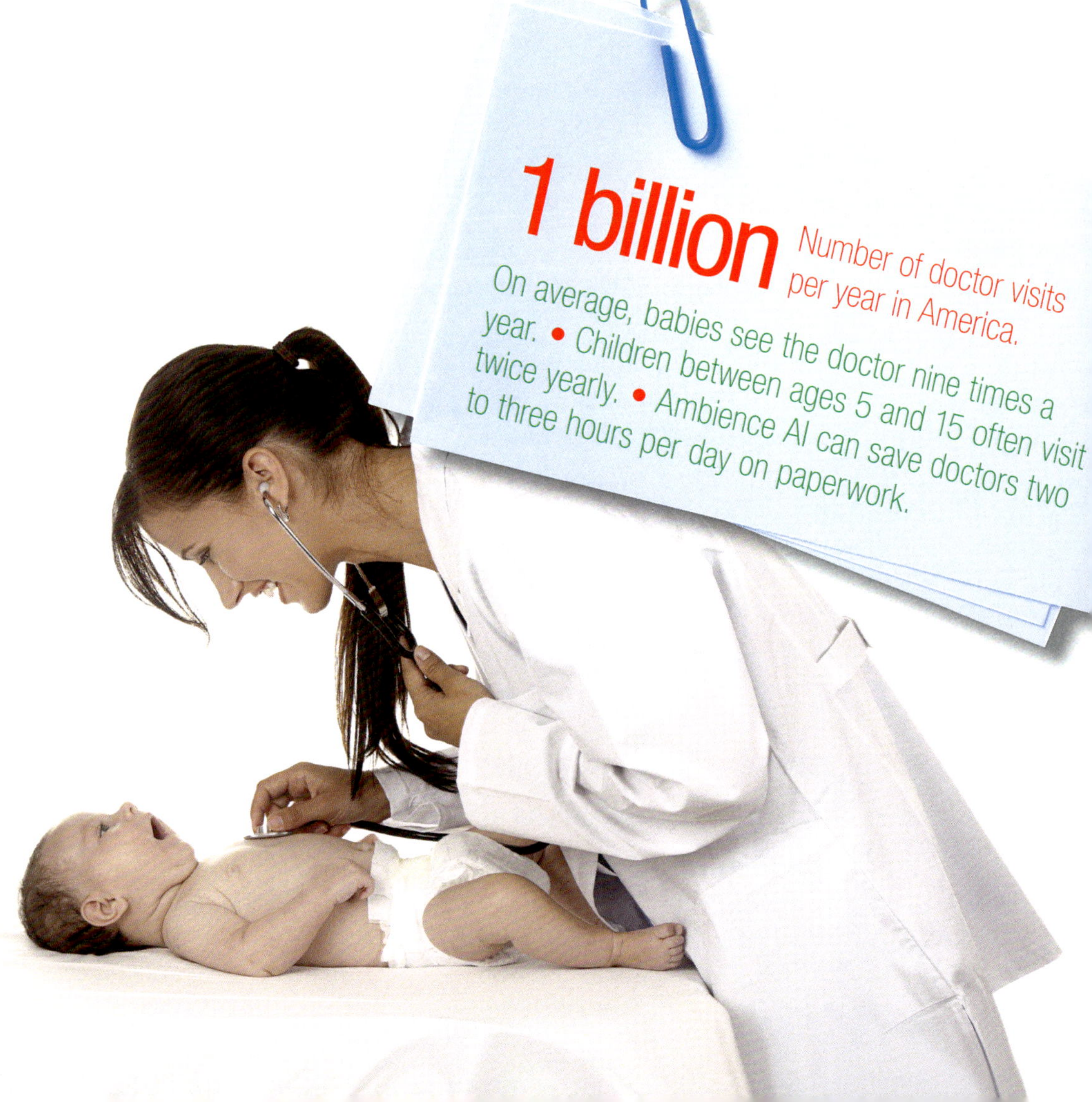

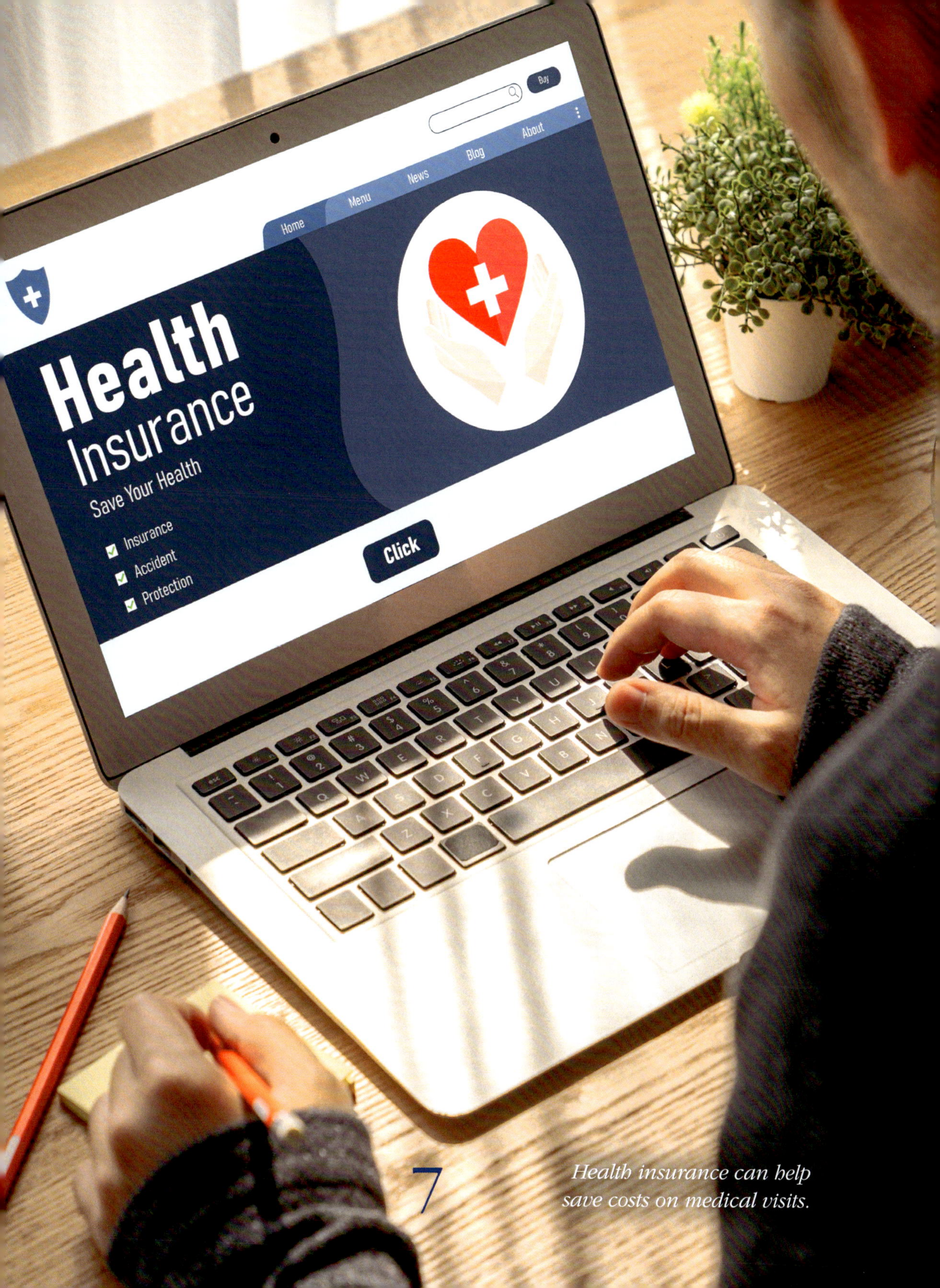

Health insurance can help save costs on medical visits.

AI Can Screen *for Cancer*

2

Cancer is still a mystery to doctors. There are many unanswered questions. Why do people get cancer? What is the best way to treat it? How do we stop it from coming back? Missing an early sign can be deadly. Some people live far away from high-quality medical care. And there are many types of cancer. One treatment does not work on all types.

AI can help save lives. It is already used in both cancer research and care. It looks at tumors. This is a lump of cells that do not grow normally. It **predicts** what type of cancer cells might form. It also finds cancer cells.

ChatGPT can be used on smartphones.

Researchers at Harvard are working on their own AI. It is called CHIEF.AI. It is similar to ChatGPT. Their tool can perform a variety of different cancer-related tasks. One is looking

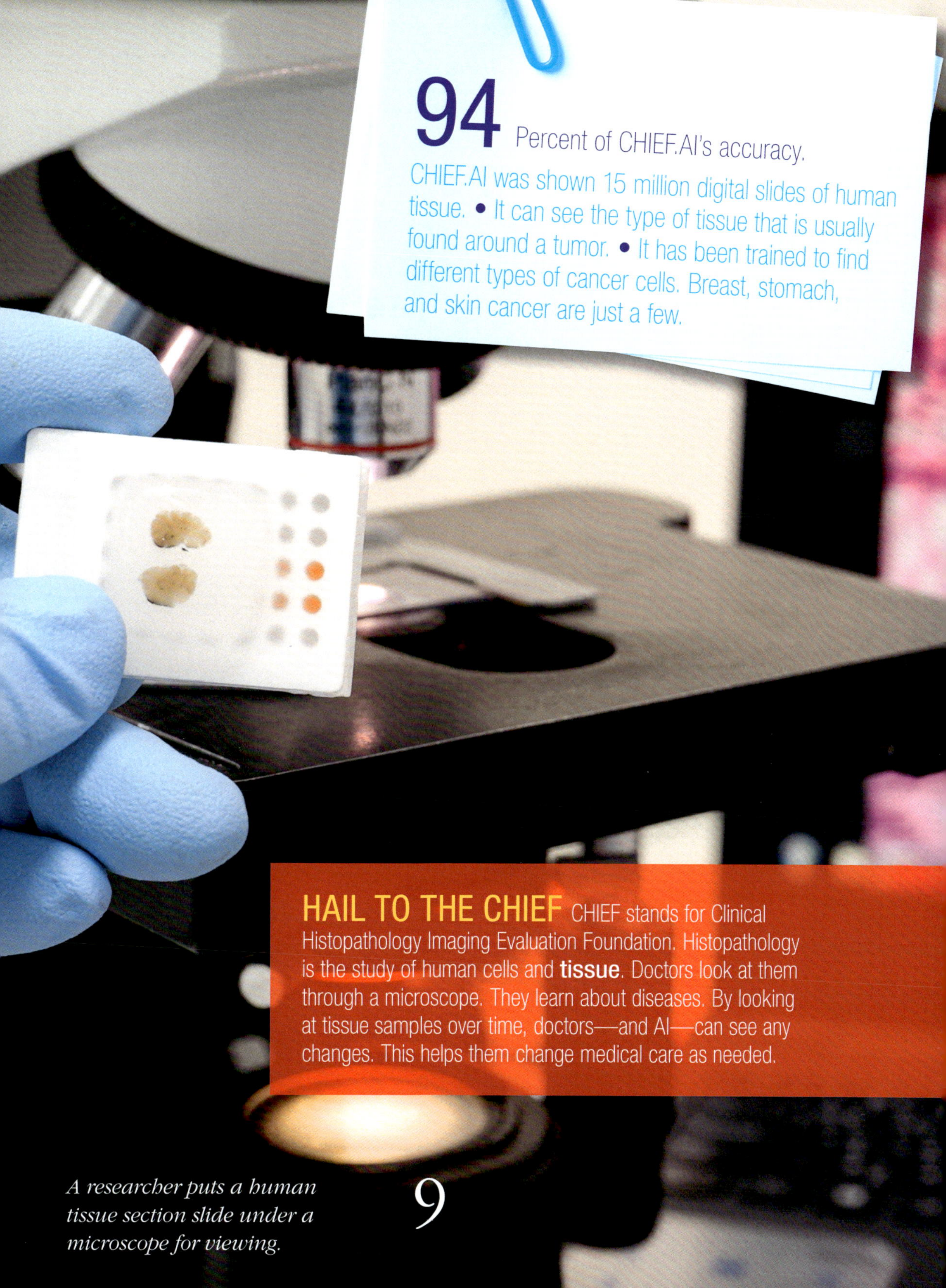

94 Percent of CHIEF.AI's accuracy.

CHIEF.AI was shown 15 million digital slides of human tissue. • It can see the type of tissue that is usually found around a tumor. • It has been trained to find different types of cancer cells. Breast, stomach, and skin cancer are just a few.

HAIL TO THE CHIEF CHIEF stands for Clinical Histopathology Imaging Evaluation Foundation. Histopathology is the study of human cells and **tissue**. Doctors look at them through a microscope. They learn about diseases. By looking at tissue samples over time, doctors—and AI—can see any changes. This helps them change medical care as needed.

A researcher puts a human tissue section slide under a microscope for viewing.

at different treatments. Another includes comparing them to other patient studies.

Before CHIEF.AI, doctors spent hours studying. They looked at tissue samples and body scans. They looked for tumors or other things that were out of place. They may be unsure about what they see. Or they might not be familiar with a patient's medical history. They could ask the patient to come back in to take new samples or scans. But this is time-consuming and expensive. CHIEF.AI has already looked at millions of images. It knows exactly what to look for. It is quicker and more accurate than a person.

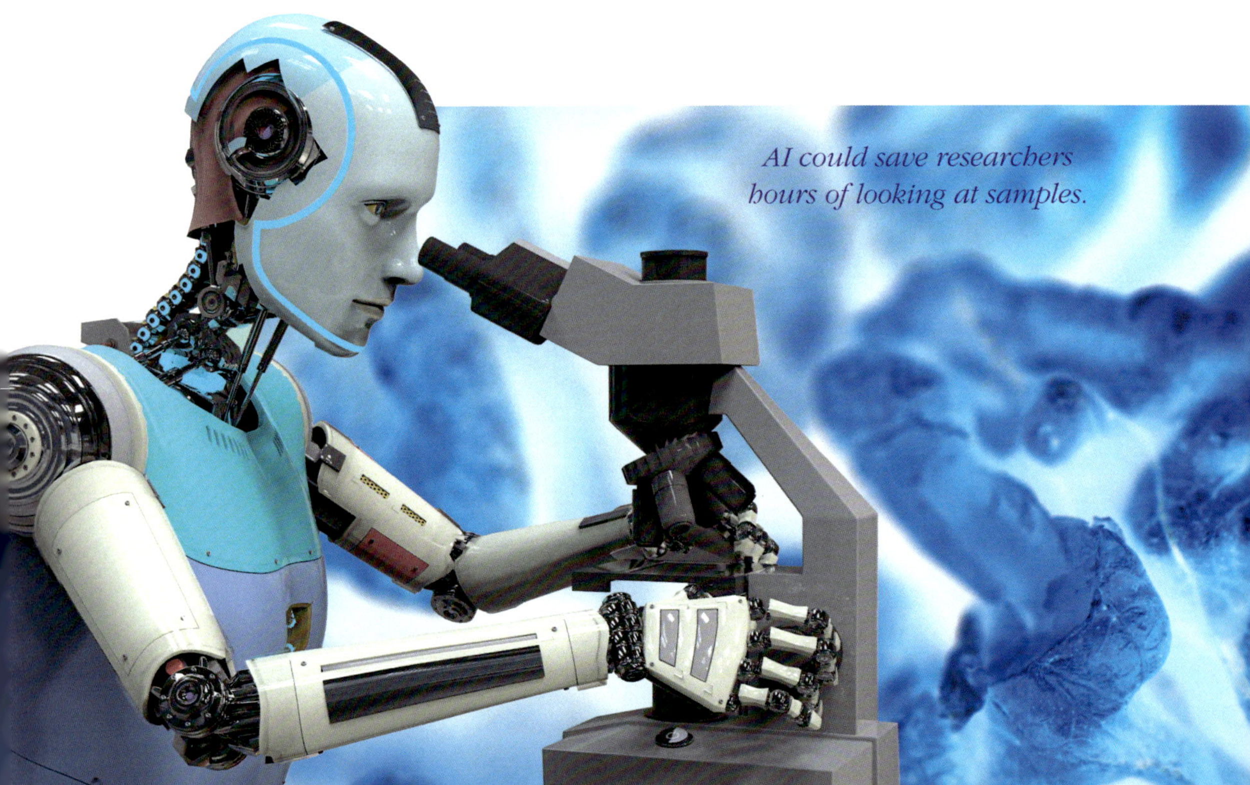

AI could save researchers hours of looking at samples.

AI Chatbots Are Here *to Talk*

3

Mental health problems can occur at any time. But getting in touch with a therapist after hours can be hard. There might not be an office in **rural** areas. Some people can't afford the care. Others are afraid of being seen and judged. All these things keep people from getting support.

AI chatbots could be the answer. They are available 24/7. People do not need appointments. Mental health apps are easy to download. People around the world can use them. And they do not have to leave their home. Privacy is important. People are more likely to talk about personal issues. A chatbot may help them feel safe from judgement too.

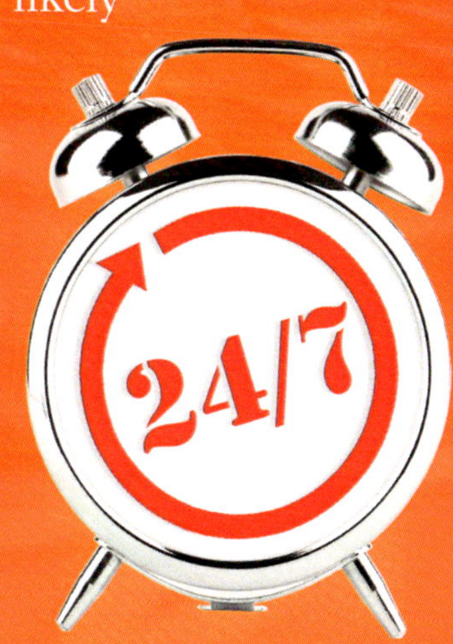

Chatbots send users daily reminders. They can check in every day. This keeps people accountable. They can easily log activities and moods. Over time, they can compare data. The bot sends reminders for exercise and appointments.

Chatbots are good for support. They can offer basic treatment plans. But they cannot identify emergency situations. They work best when used with a human counselor. They can create a more personalized experience.

17 Percent of kids aged 6 to 17 who experience a mental health disorder.
Only around half of these kids get treatment. • Women are more likely to seek mental health care than men. • Common mental health disorders are anxiety and depression.

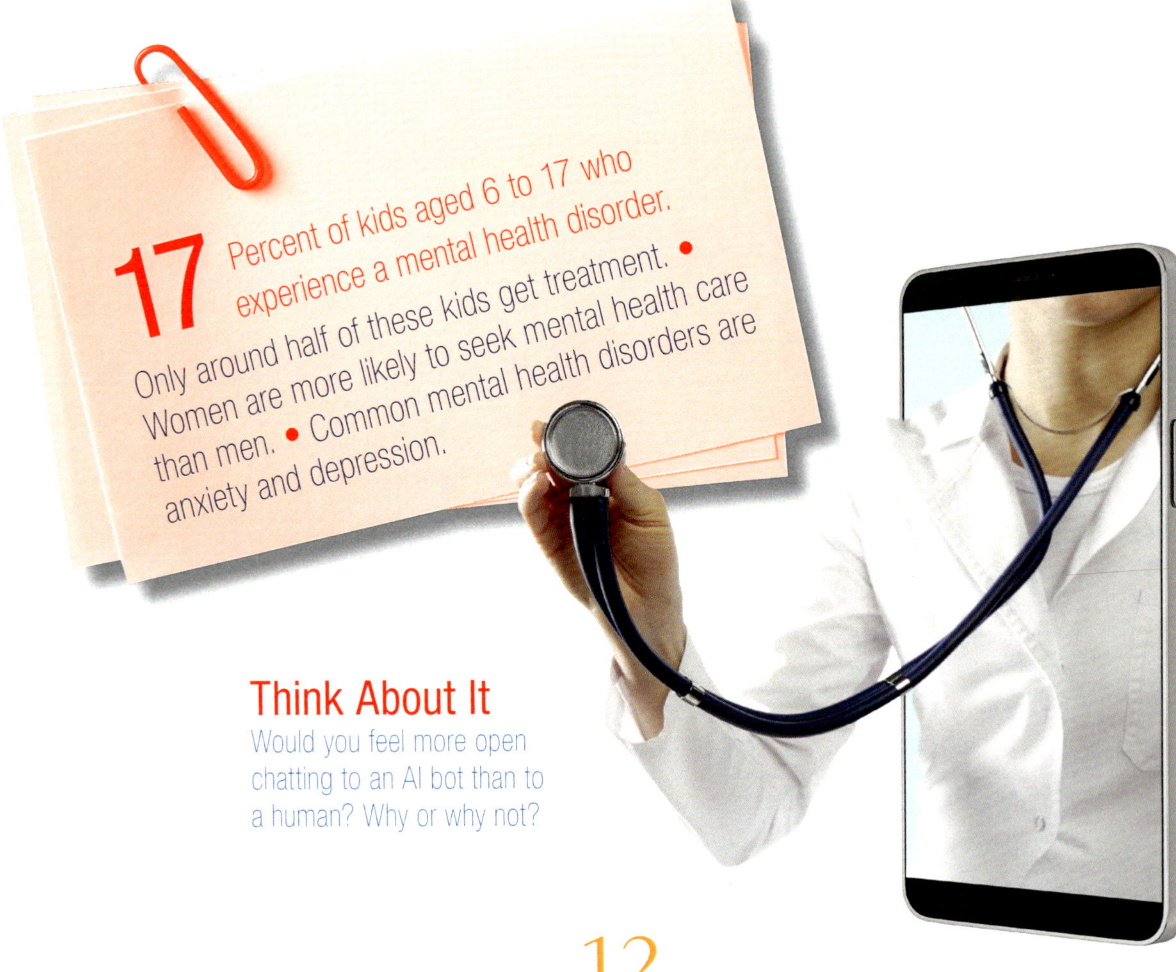

Think About It

Would you feel more open chatting to an AI bot than to a human? Why or why not?

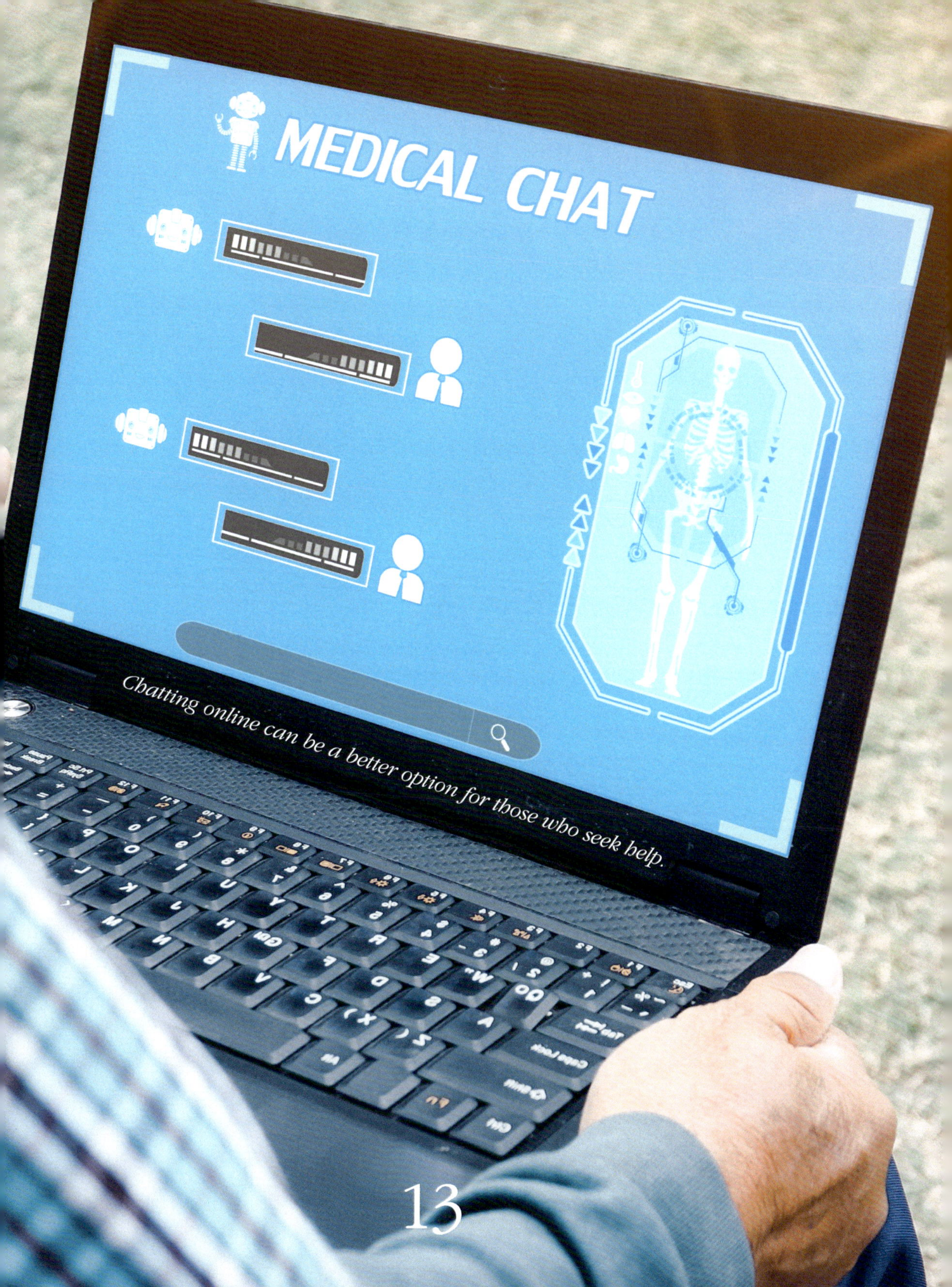

Chatting online can be a better option for those who seek help.

One More Lap Around the *AI Track*

4

Athletes push their bodies and minds as far as possible. This can lead to big gains. It can also cause injuries. Some injuries are easy to see. Others are not. Common injuries are hairline fractures, muscle tears, and concussions. These can take time to **diagnose**.

With AI's help, athletes can learn what therapies will work best with their injury. The National Football League (NFL) uses an AI tool called Digital Athlete. It views the player's entire career. It helps create personalized training and recovery plans. It also tells teams which players are at high risk for injury.

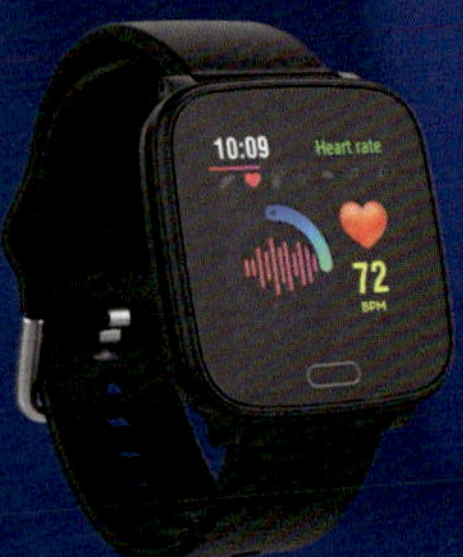

Smartwatches can track heart rate and sleep patterns.

Athletes also use AI to help train. They can avoid injuries before they happen. Tracking apps such as Ochy and Uplift record **biometrics**. These are things like heart rate, muscle activity, and hormone levels. AI can

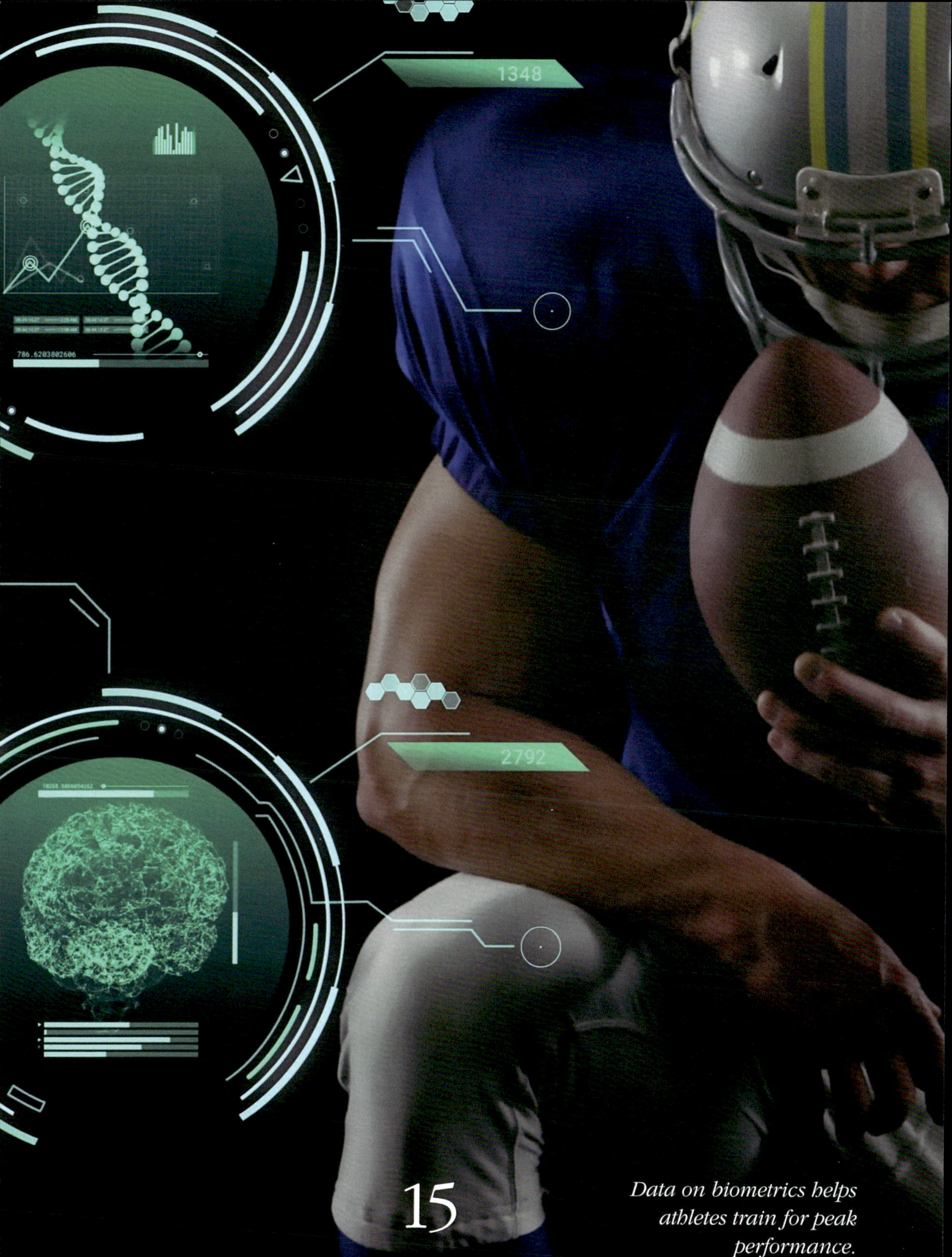

Data on biometrics helps athletes train for peak performance.

also figure out the best time to work out. It knows how long a person needs to warm up or rest. It knows if they are at risk of pushing themselves too far.

AI adapts to a person. It looks at their fitness levels, goals, and lifestyle. Then it makes a custom plan. It adjusts plans quickly with feedback. All the information can be shared with coaches and doctors. The whole team stays up to date. This improves the athlete's progress.

8.6 million Number of sports-related injuries in the United States every year.
This includes more than 775,000 children under the age of 14. • Almost one-third of childhood injuries are sports-related. • Sprains and strains are the most common.

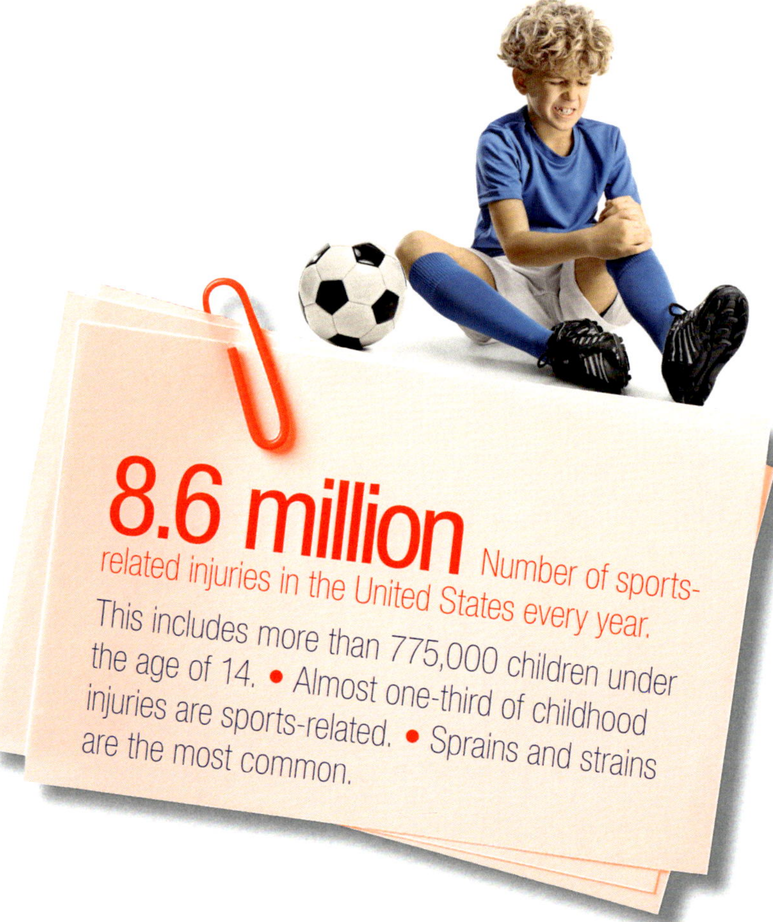

GAMES WIDE OPEN The 2024 Paris Olympics fully embraced AI. There was an AI assistant that helped athletes remember rules or find their way. There was technology to protect athletes against negative social media comments. AI cameras were used for security.

Paging Doctor AI *to Surgery*

5

Robot-assisted surgery has been around for decades. Robots help surgeons work faster. The doctors can work in more comfort too. Robots can make the same movements over and over again. They are very precise. However, they can't make decisions. And they can't adapt to new situations. That's where AI comes in.

Doctors, robots, and AI all have their own strengths. They use knowledge in different ways. They have different skill sets. When combined, surgery can be safer. Robots can take on simpler tasks. This saves time. The robot follows a doctor's orders. It also follows safety rules. If something goes wrong, a doctor can step in and take over.

The da Vinci Surgical System is a medical AI robot. In 2024, it watched hundreds of videos. These were recorded by surgeons wearing special wrist cameras.

The videos showed three skills. One was using a needle. The second was lifting body tissue. The third was sewing up a wound.

The da Vinci robot copied what it saw in the videos. Eventually, it was able to do all the movements. With practice, it could do them as well as the surgeons. It even learned new things on its own. For example, if it dropped a needle, it picked it up and kept going.

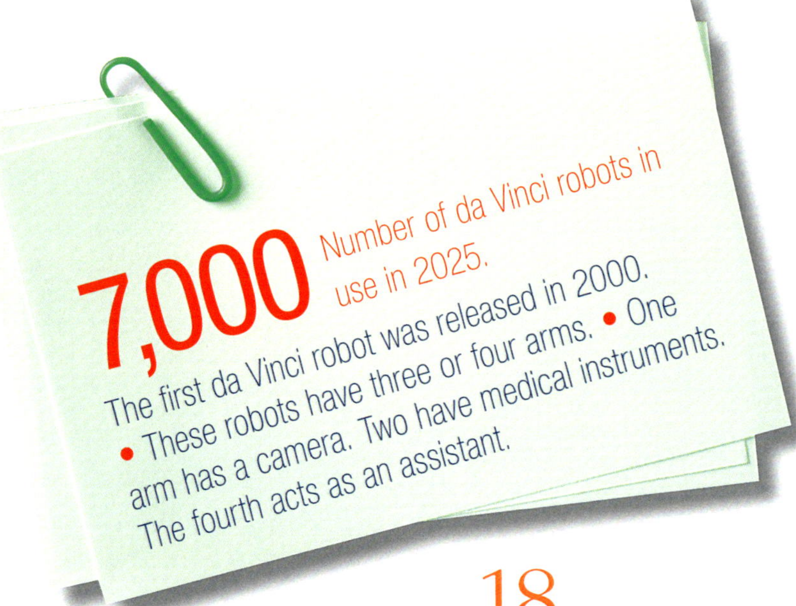

7,000 Number of da Vinci robots in use in 2025.

The first da Vinci robot was released in 2000. • These robots have three or four arms. • One arm has a camera. Two have medical instruments. The fourth acts as an assistant.

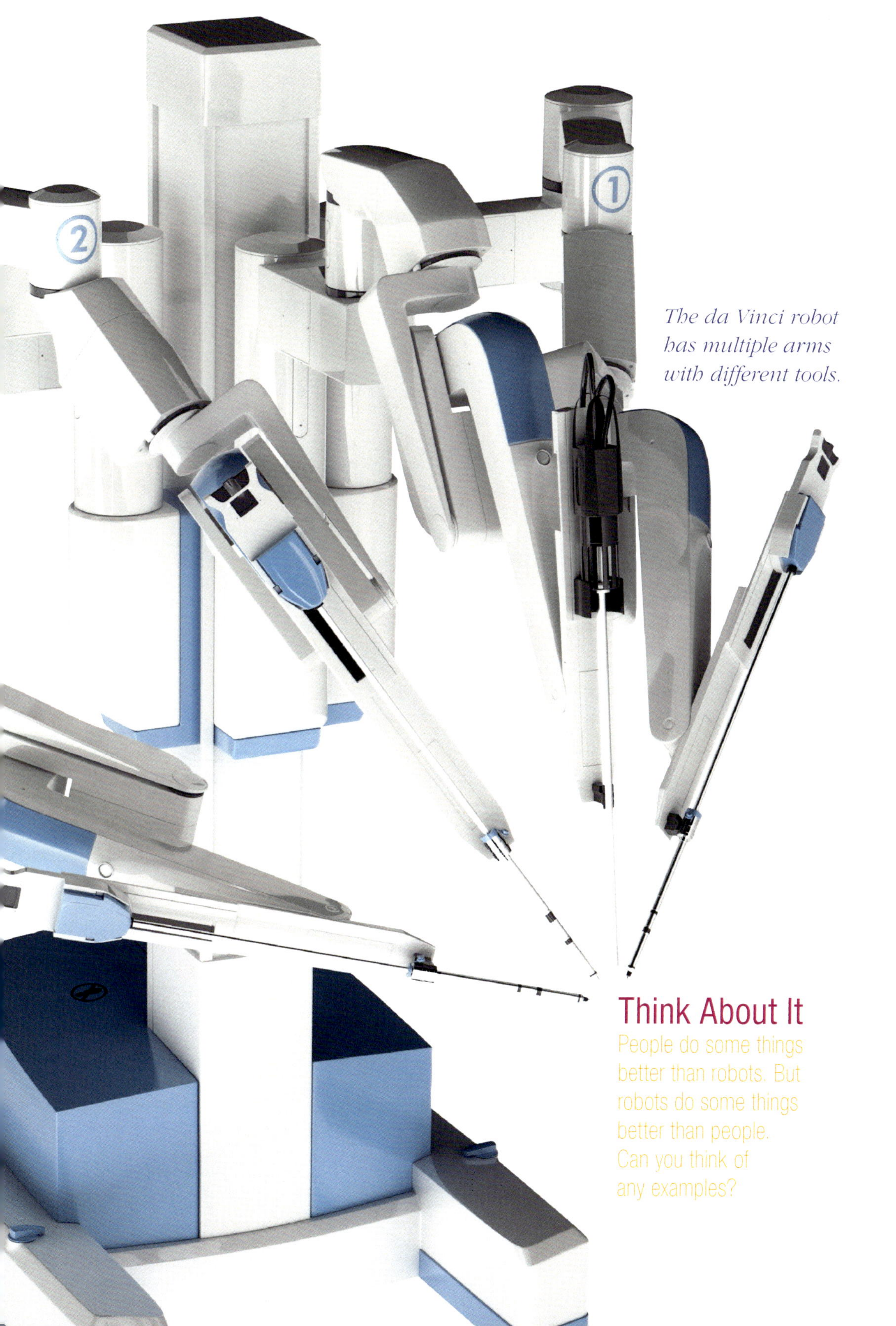

The da Vinci robot has multiple arms with different tools.

Think About It

People do some things better than robots. But robots do some things better than people. Can you think of any examples?

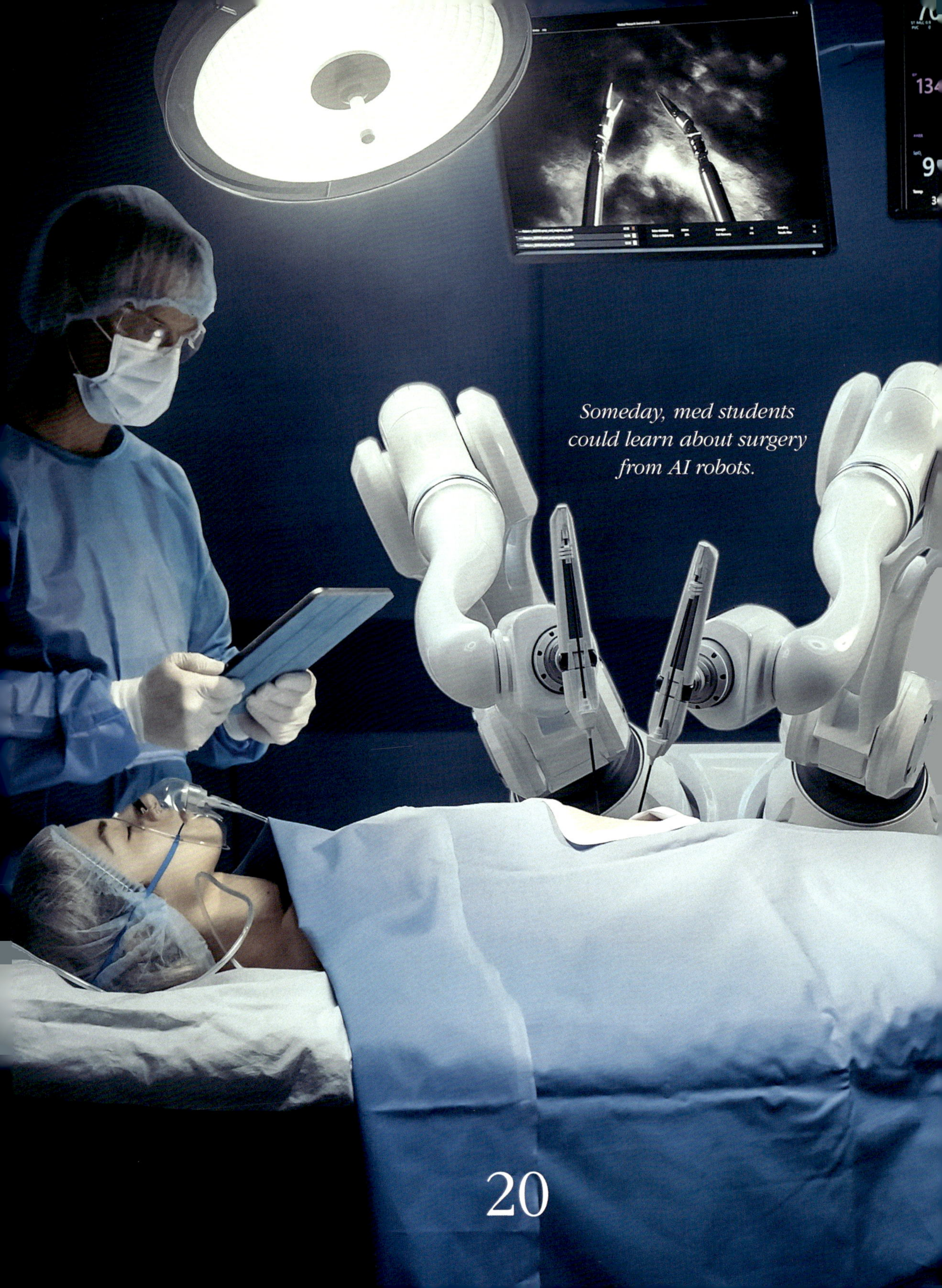

Someday, med students could learn about surgery from AI robots.

Training Doctors and Nurses *with AI*

6

It takes a long time to become a doctor or a nurse. Without teachers, medical students have no one to learn from. The more teachers there are, the more students can learn. But what if the teachers were AI?

In March 2023, ChatGPT took the United States Medical Licensing Exam (USMLE). It passed. It hadn't even studied for the test! By April 2024, it was able to score as high as human doctors. The results scared some people. They wondered if AI was on its way to replacing humans. But medical educators began thinking ahead.

Harvard Medical School started with a basic course. It taught about AI in healthcare. Now, they have a full PhD program. It is called Artificial Intelligence in Medicine. Students work with AI researchers. They build new tools for the medical field.

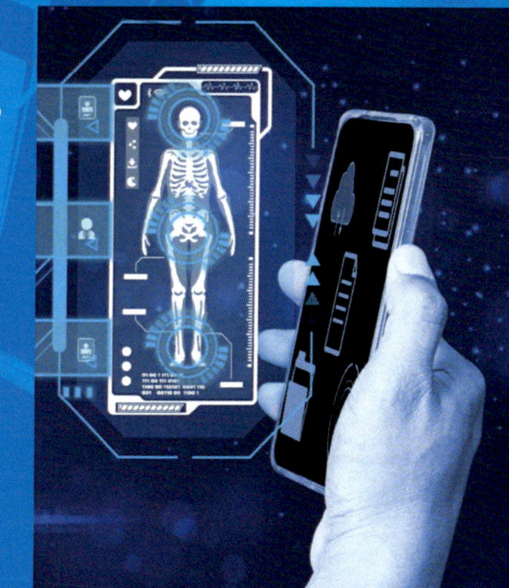

AI helps students learn the most up-to-date information. They also get a unique perspective. They can take a deeper look at the way they see the world.

AI has one big downfall. It is only as good as the information it's given. This can feed into **biases**. Students must be extra careful. They should watch for any biases or wrong information.

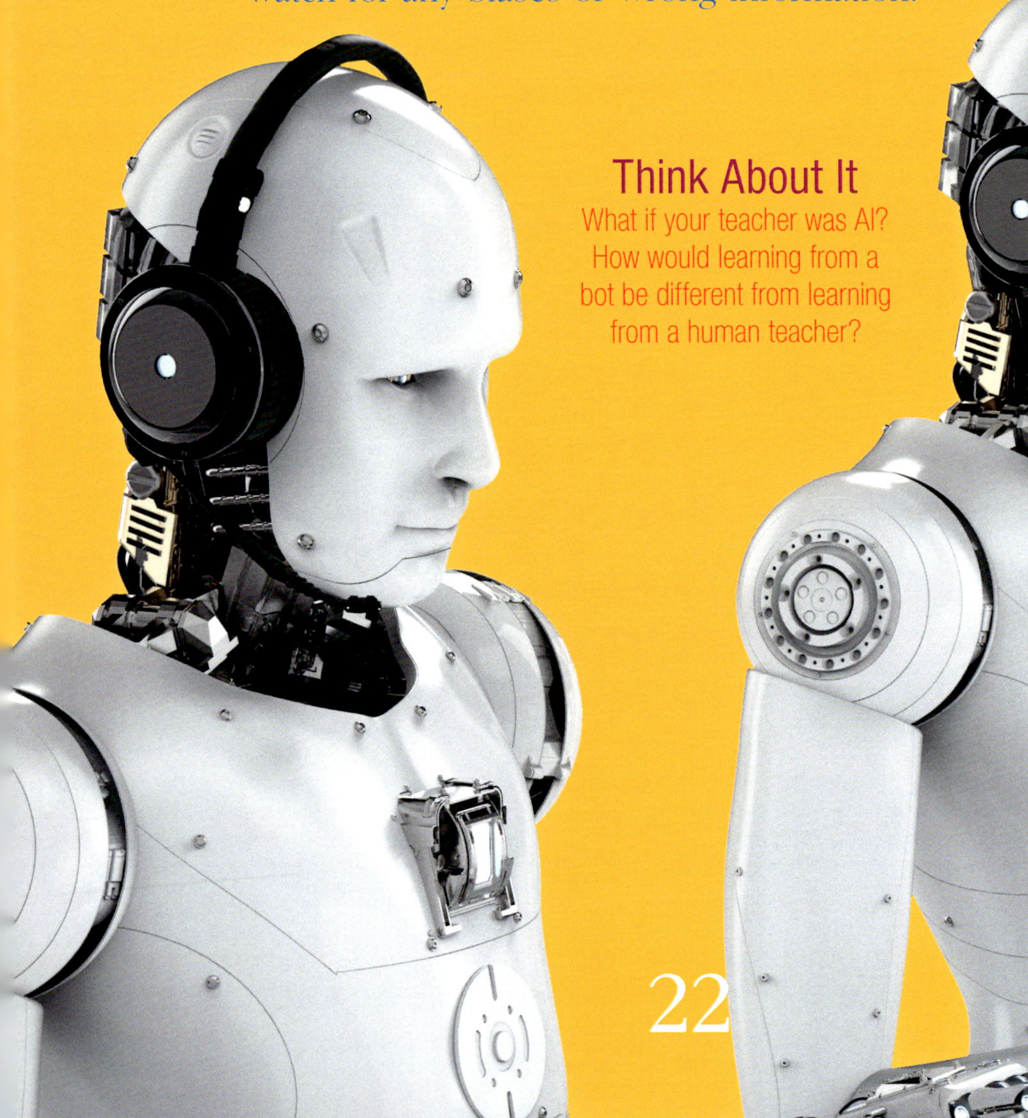

Think About It

What if your teacher was AI? How would learning from a bot be different from learning from a human teacher?

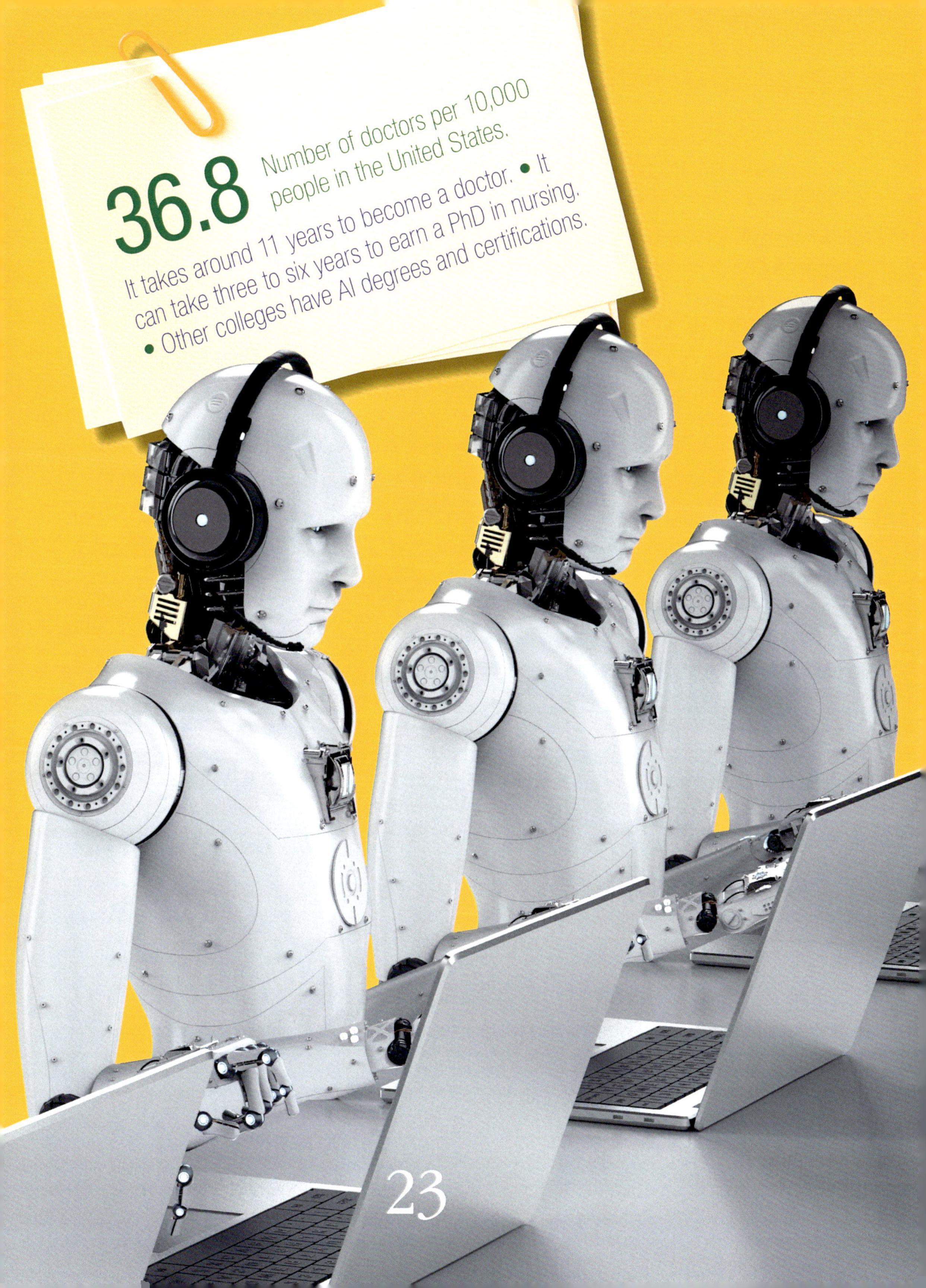

36.8 Number of doctors per 10,000 people in the United States.

It takes around 11 years to become a doctor. • It can take three to six years to earn a PhD in nursing. • Other colleges have AI degrees and certifications.

AI Helps Patients Take *Their Medicine*

7 Some people need to take medicine every day. Others need to take it at certain times. They might need to take it under very specific conditions. It can be hard to remember. Sometimes it is painful or unpleasant. People simply do not want to do it.

Scientists at MIT and the University of Galway worked together. They created an AI **implant**. It gives people their medicine. It is painless and blends in perfectly. The person doesn't even remember it is there.

The implants are called soft robotics. They are flexible and tiny. They are inspired by human skin. This idea is called biomimicry. It models technology after nature.

Some implants attach under the skin. Others are inserted into the body. They may stick to organs. Other ones are swallowed. They stay in the digestive system.

HERE FOR PICKUP

AI is also being used by **pharmacists**. Some drugs do not work well together. AI can alert pharmacists to any bad reactions. It can also check patients' refill history. People who miss a pickup are flagged. They might not be taking their medicine the right way.

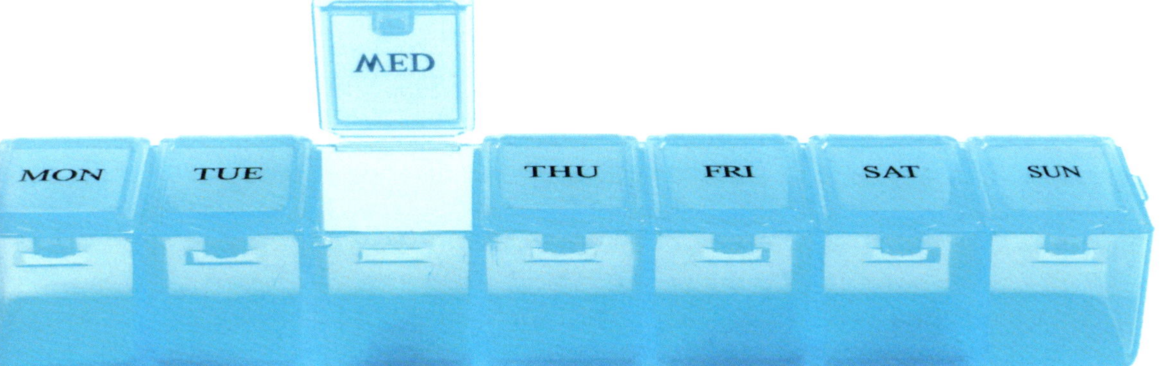

Each type can sense when the body needs more of its drug. It releases the correct amount.

The human body does not like unfamiliar things. It tends to reject anything that does not belong. It also creates scar tissue. Scar tissue makes it harder to give medication. Soft robots sense when scar tissue is forming. They move and change shape to prevent it.

65 Percent of US adults who take at least one prescription drug each day.
Some medicines need to be taken at the same time every day. • Some work better at different times of the day. • Missing a dose is bad for a person's health.

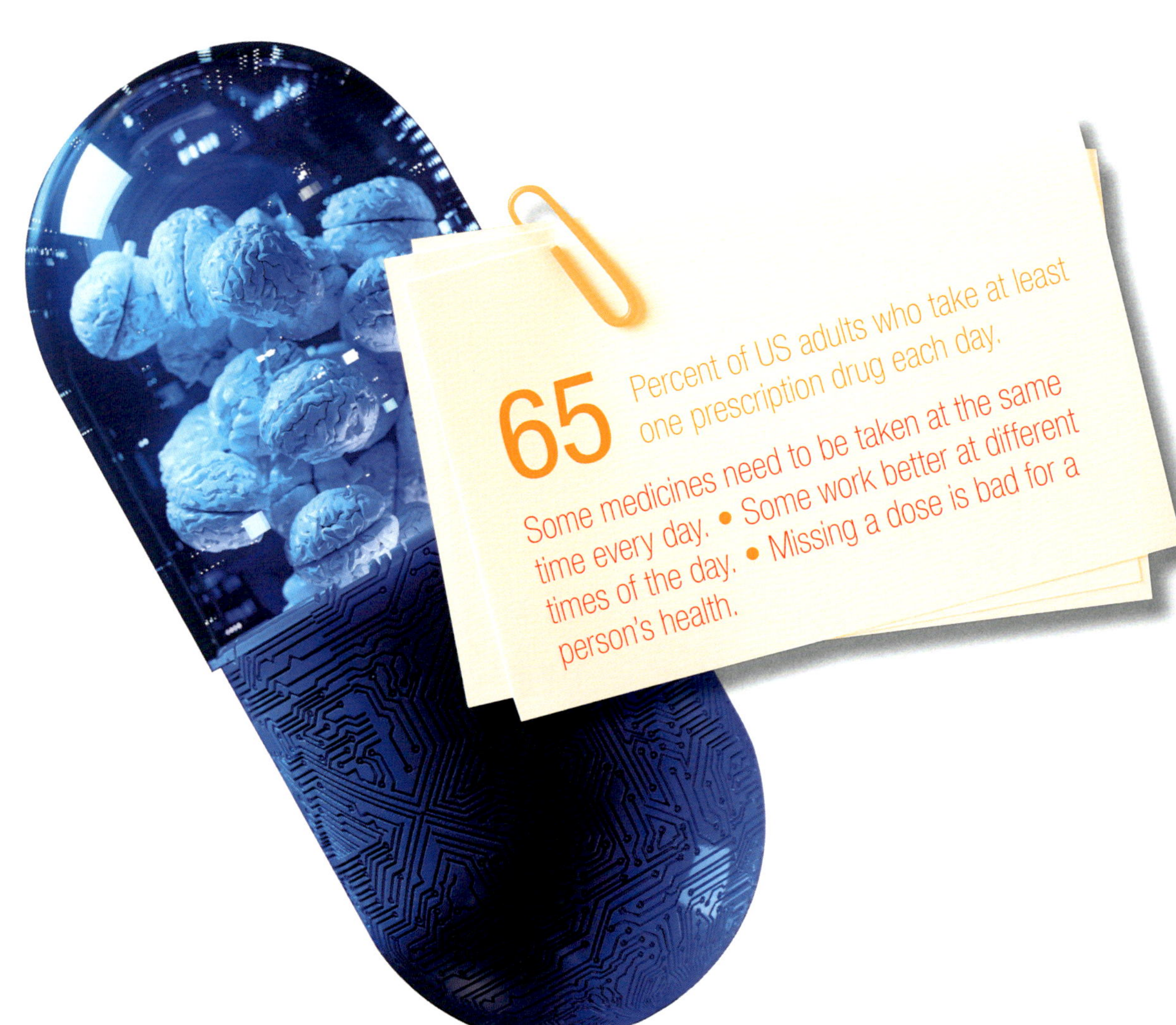

AI Takes Emergency Calls *and Saves Lives*

8

In an emergency, every minute counts. The moment an accident happens, the clock starts. Lives are at stake until help arrives. The injured person may have a short time until they die. Emergency medical services (EMS) can slow this clock. The moment they arrive, they help the injured. They get them stable enough to go to the hospital. Each second matters.

AI can help EMS workers. It can predict the need for **critical** care. It can show who needs care first. It can also warn emergency rooms that there are patients coming. That way, they know what to prepare for.

In 2023, an emergency center in the Netherlands tested out AI. They noticed AI made decisions faster than a human. It could see where ambulances were being sent by other call-takers at the same time. In all, AI saved EMS about seven weeks of work!

One AI tool is called Corti.ai. It listens to the caller's **vital signs**. It can detect the possibility of heart attack. If it believes the caller is at risk, it alerts a human operator. The operator tells the caller to seek out emergency care. It increases the survival rate by 20 percent.

One issue with 911 callers is poor sound quality. An AI system can **transcribe** these calls. It highlights keywords often used during medical emergencies. Another issue is getting too many calls at once. This happens during disasters. Chatbots can respond to more than one caller at once. They send more difficult calls to humans.

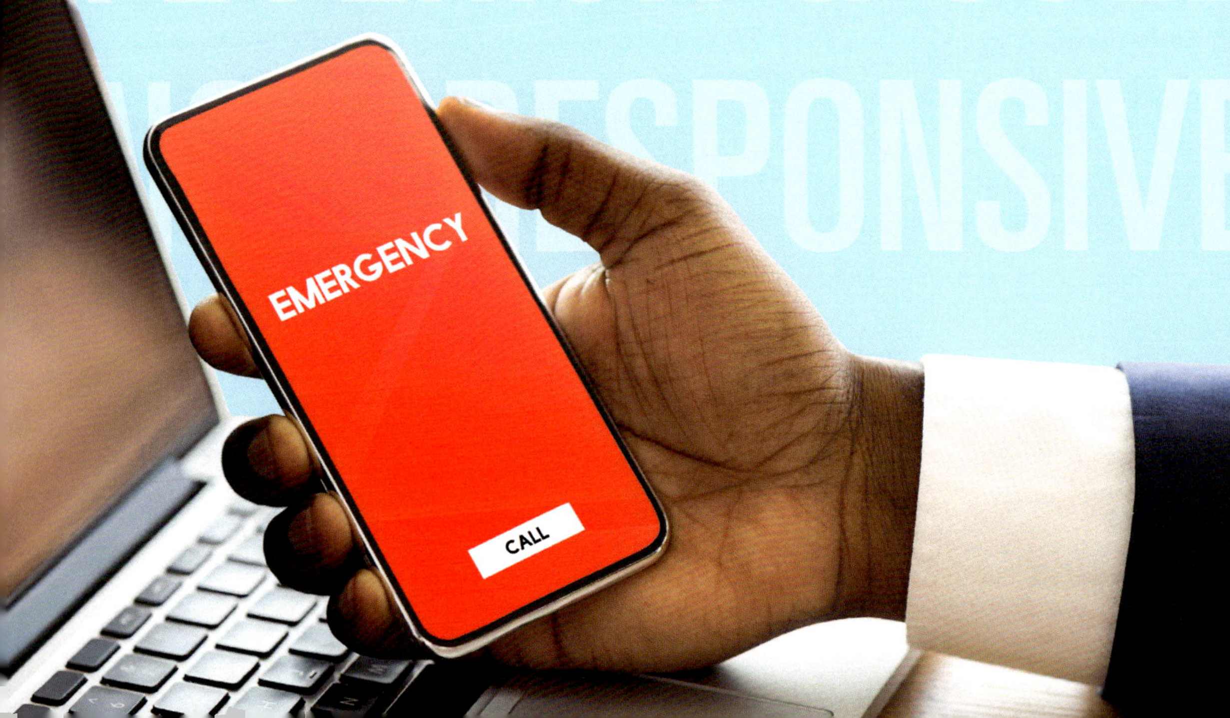

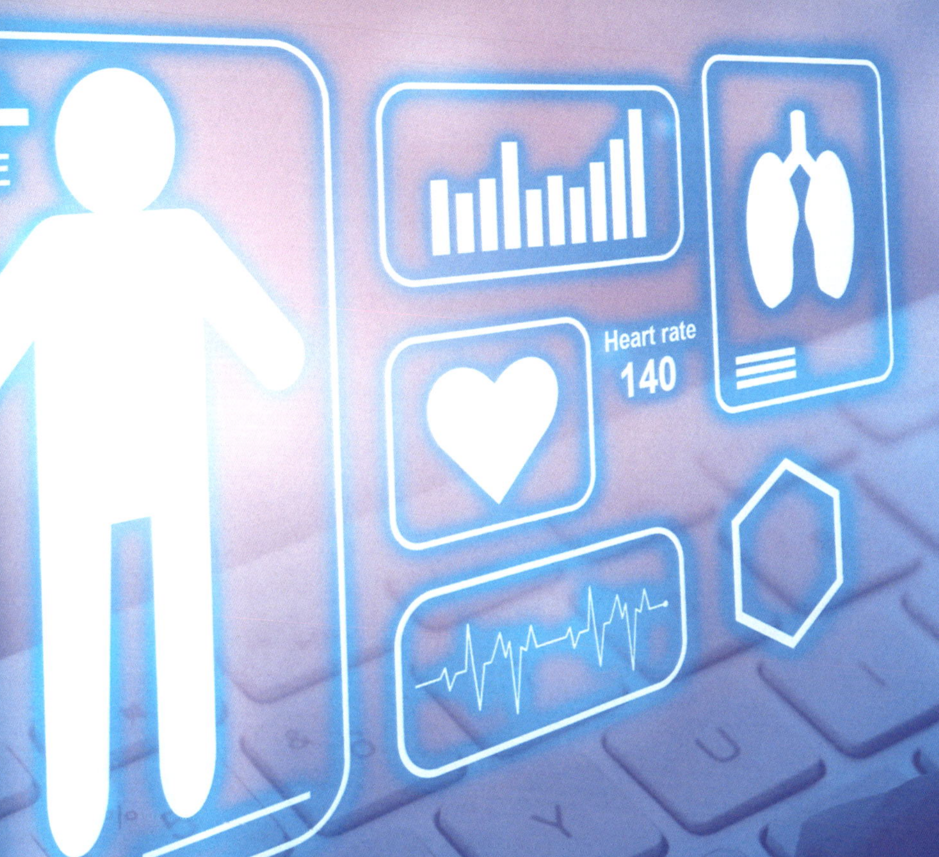

163 Average number of minutes patients spent in emergency rooms in 2024.

Emergency room visits can cost $1,200 or more. • Using AI could lower costs and save patients money. • AI may be more efficient at communicating during emergencies.

AI can help emergency centers respond to calls more quickly.

AI Helps Rural Patients Get *Better Treatment*

9

Most Americans live 10 miles (16 kilometers) or less from a hospital. For people in rural areas, it may be two or three times that distance. Rural hospitals may have limited resources. They may also cost more and have a shortage of providers. Due to this, more and more rural hospitals are closing every year.

Using AI and **telemedicine** can help. One tool is Ada. It is a smartphone app for patients. Ada has a Condition Library. Patients can list their symptoms. They can review health changes over time. The library helps them understand what they might have. It finds them the necessary care. Ada can also make sure patients go to the right hospital for treatment.

The University of Michigan is leading another AI-powered program. It is on wheels! A van could drive to patients.

Human healthcare workers would ride along. These would be nurses or family doctors. The van's AI is called VIGIL. It would help them diagnose injuries and illnesses. It would guide them through unfamiliar procedures. VIGIL would have the ability to learn. It could adapt to best serve its patients and staff. It would bring hospitals directly to the people.

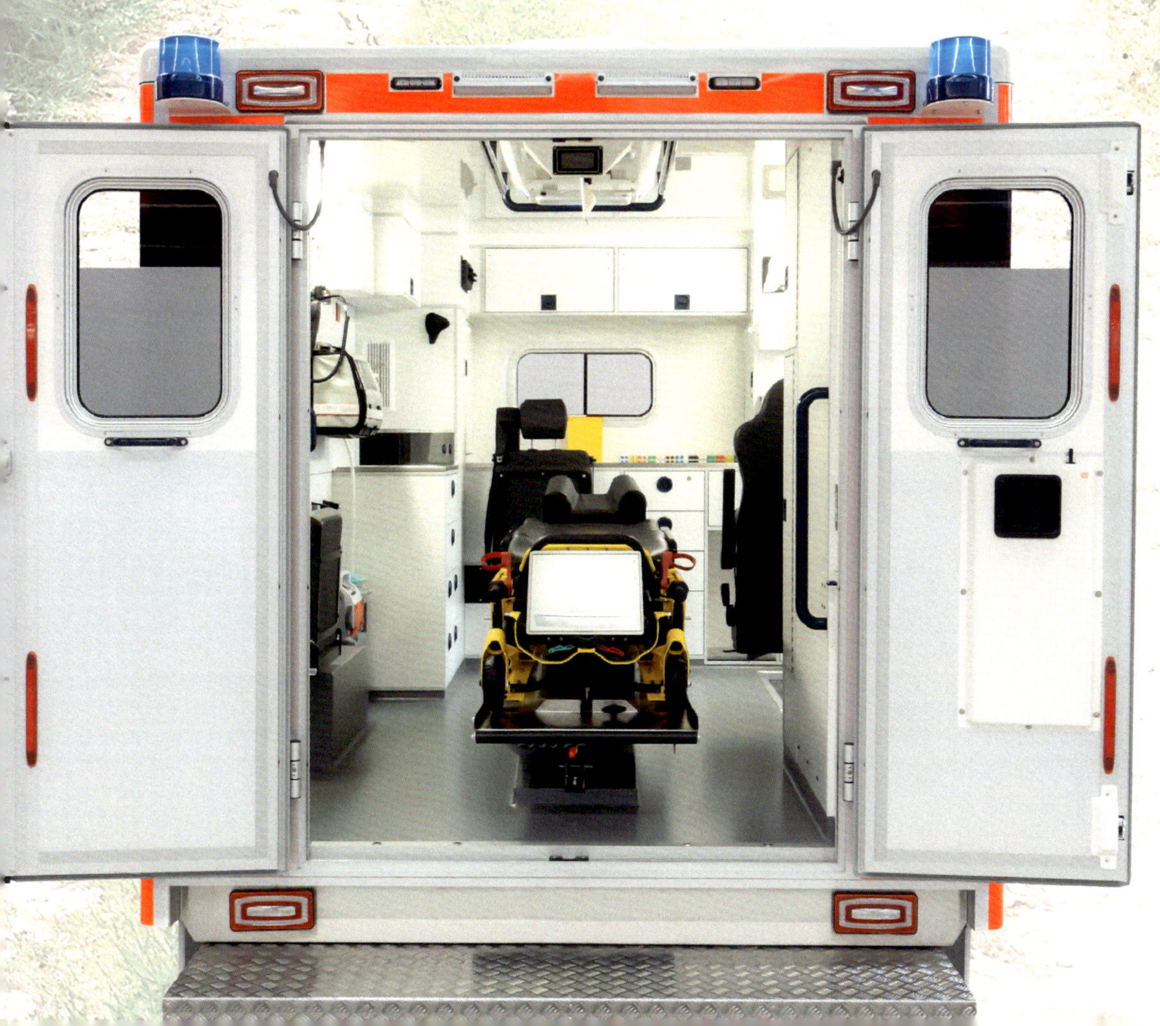

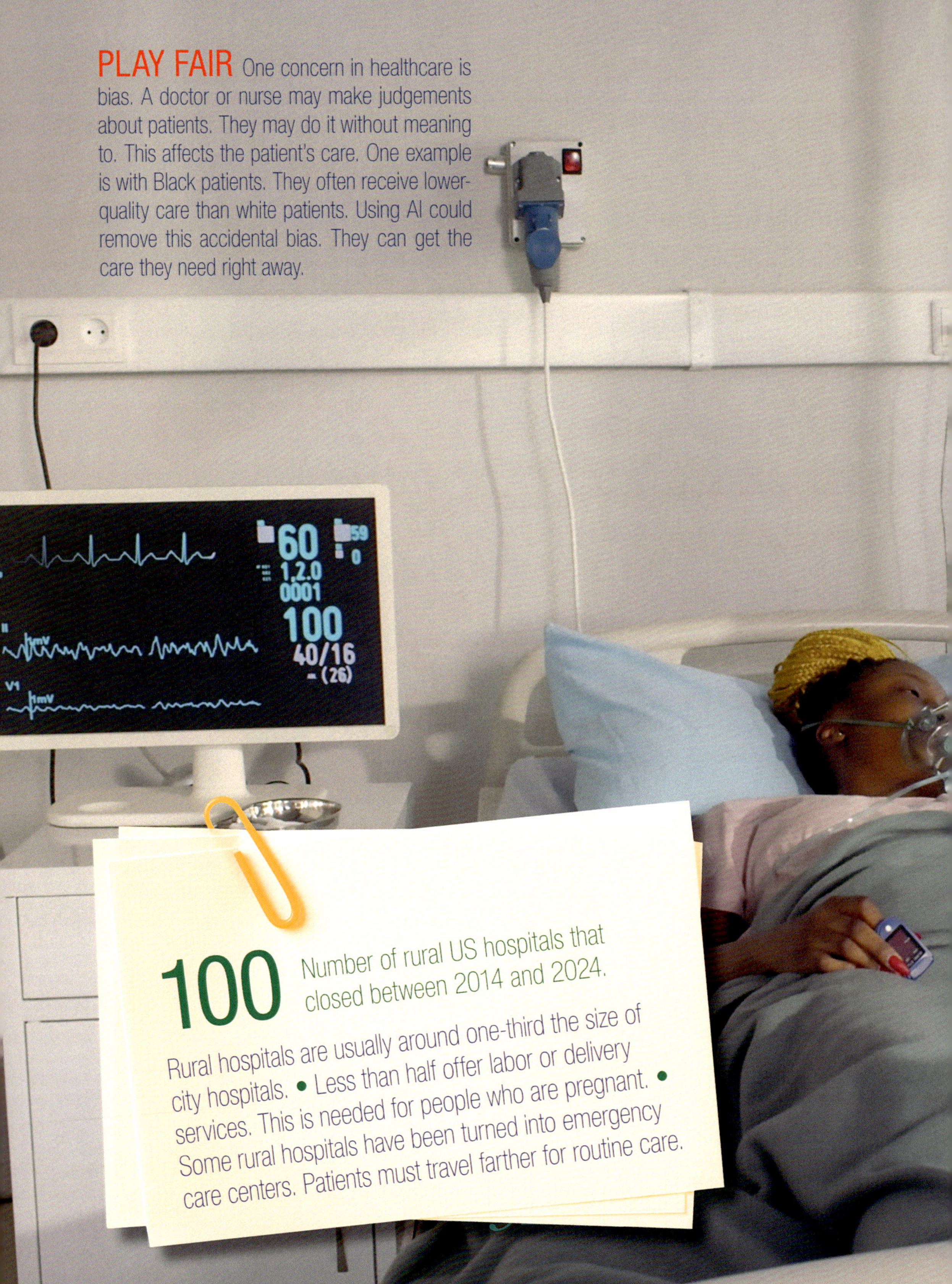

PLAY FAIR One concern in healthcare is bias. A doctor or nurse may make judgements about patients. They may do it without meaning to. This affects the patient's care. One example is with Black patients. They often receive lower-quality care than white patients. Using AI could remove this accidental bias. They can get the care they need right away.

100 Number of rural US hospitals that closed between 2014 and 2024.

Rural hospitals are usually around one-third the size of city hospitals. • Less than half offer labor or delivery services. This is needed for people who are pregnant. • Some rural hospitals have been turned into emergency care centers. Patients must travel farther for routine care.

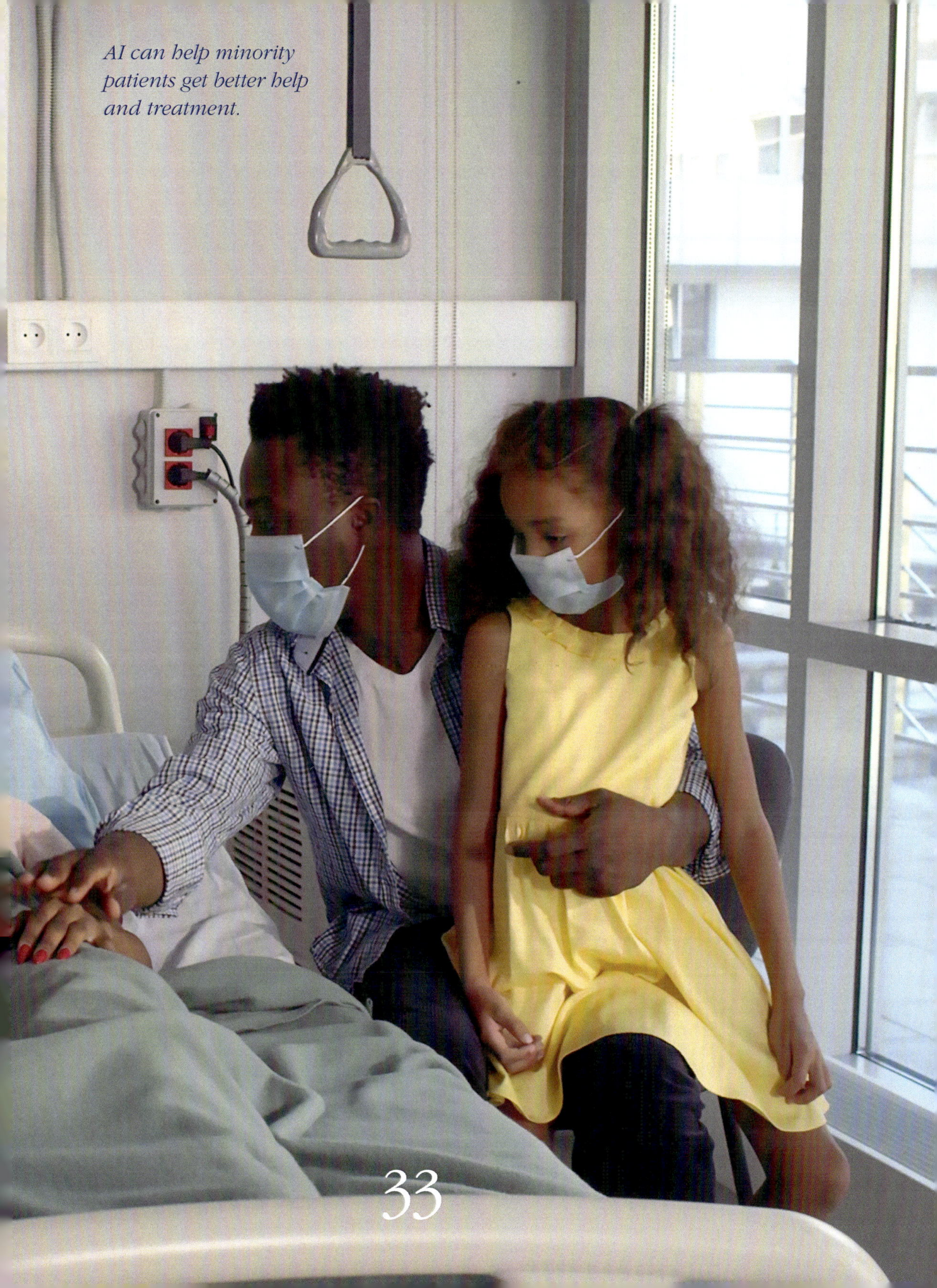

AI can help minority patients get better help and treatment.

AI Helps Doctors Get *a Better Look*

10

Digital imaging machines help doctors see inside patients. Ultrasounds and X-ray machines are two examples. Doctors look at the images before and during surgery. It helps them operate in exactly the right spot. Sometimes a patient moves during a scan. Or the machine is bumped. The image may turn out fuzzy in these cases. Then it is harder for surgeons to find the right spot. AI can fix this.

AI combines data from any and all available imaging sources. It makes a 3D model of the patient. If a patient moves, AI can show an updated view. It can also show a more detailed picture of the area. Blood cells, organs, and nerves are part of the image. Doctors can re-evaluate. They can make new decisions in real time. This shortens operating times.

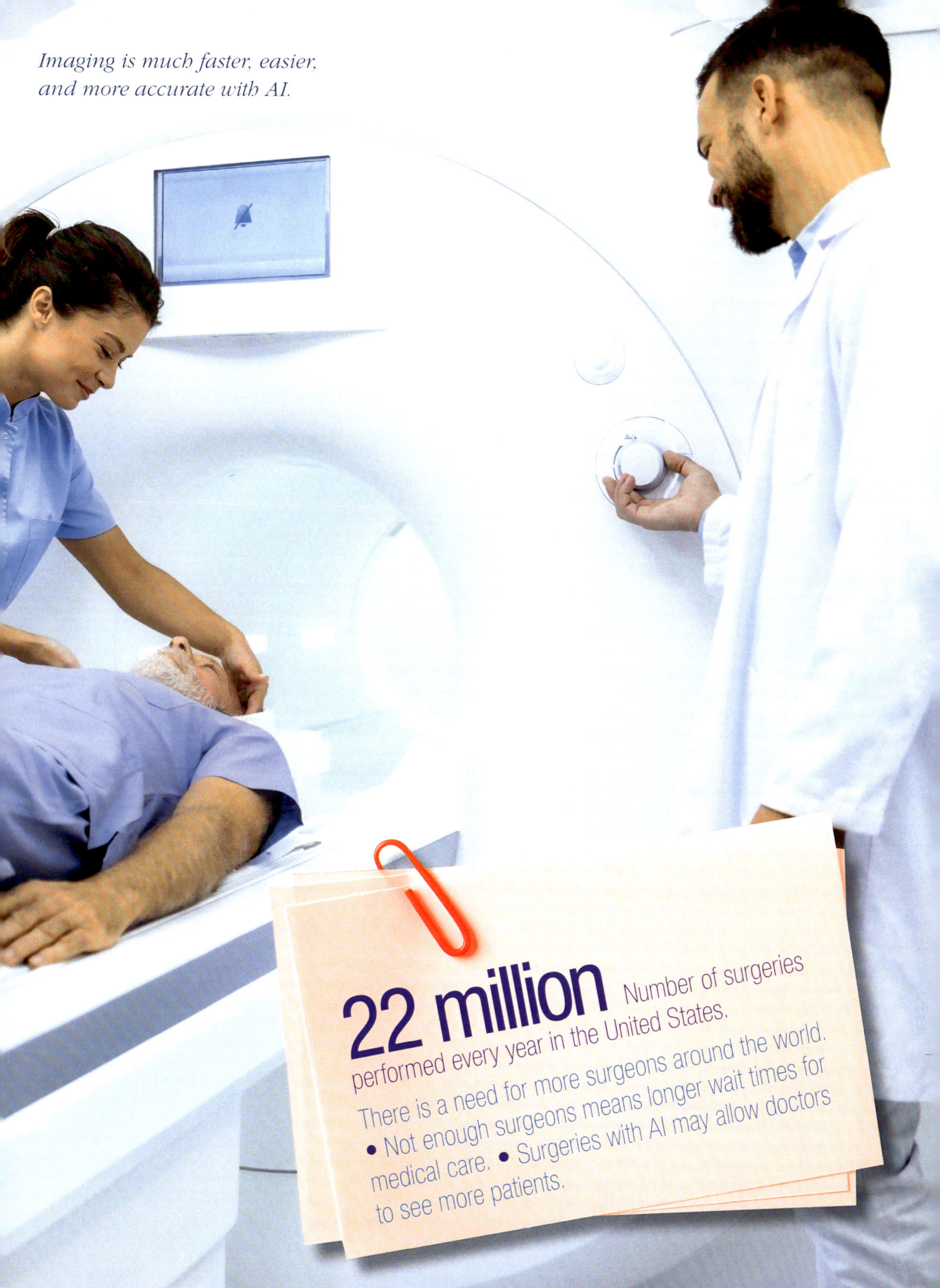

Imaging is much faster, easier, and more accurate with AI.

22 million Number of surgeries performed every year in the United States.

There is a need for more surgeons around the world. • Not enough surgeons means longer wait times for medical care. • Surgeries with AI may allow doctors to see more patients.

AI can be taught to understand what is happening during surgery. It can flag any possible risks it sees. Reducing risks can shorten the patient's healing time. It can help them avoid more surgery. This lowers costs and improves their chance for a healthy life.

There may never be a full replacement for a human surgeon. However, there are limits to how much a person can learn at once. AI can learn from thousands of real-time surgeries at once.

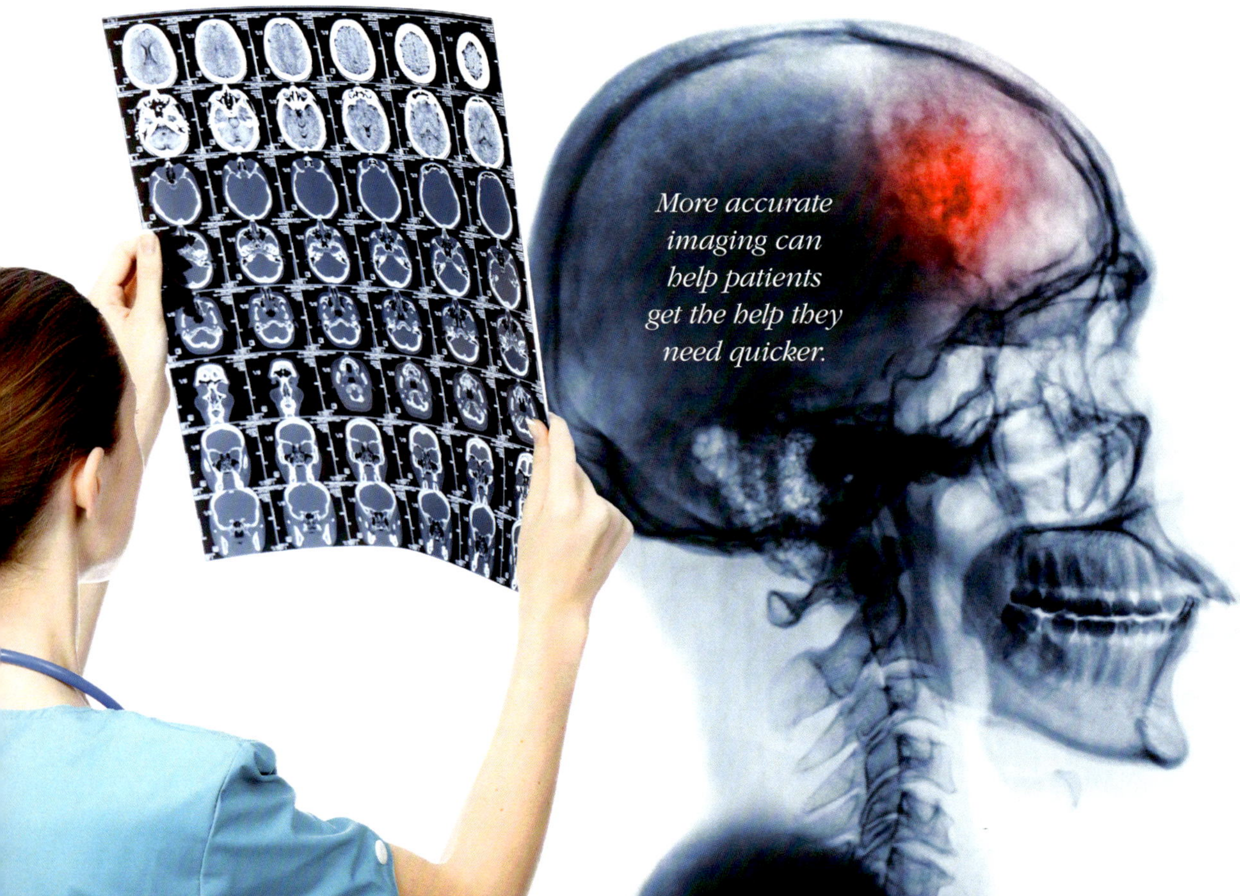

More accurate imaging can help patients get the help they need quicker.

AI Tools Can Predict *Alzheimer's Sooner*

11

Dementia is usually related with older people. It can affect anyone of any age, though. People lose the ability to remember, think clearly, or even speak. There can be many different causes. It can be caused by Alzheimer's or Parkinson's disease. People with brain damage are more likely to get dementia too.

There is still a lot doctors don't know about dementia. Many studies have collected data about the brain. Looking at it all and learning from it is a huge task. Being able to find tiny patterns sounds impossible. Using AI can help.

AI can look through the data and find patterns. It can merge data. This makes it easier to look at information from multiple sources. AI can sort patients into categories. It predicts which treatments would work best for each.

AI has already helped. Doctors can now predict Alzheimer's seven years before symptoms start. The AI tool looks for high cholesterol and osteoporosis. These are common early conditions in dementia patients.

A team at Cambridge University created another AI tool. It can predict if a patient with signs of dementia will develop Alzheimer's. It is accurate four out of five times.

12 million Number of new cases of dementia every year around the world.
Dementia was first diagnosed in 1906 by Dr. Alois Alzheimer. • Today, 55 million people around the world have dementia. • Brain scans, physical and mental tests, and physical exams can help diagnose dementia.

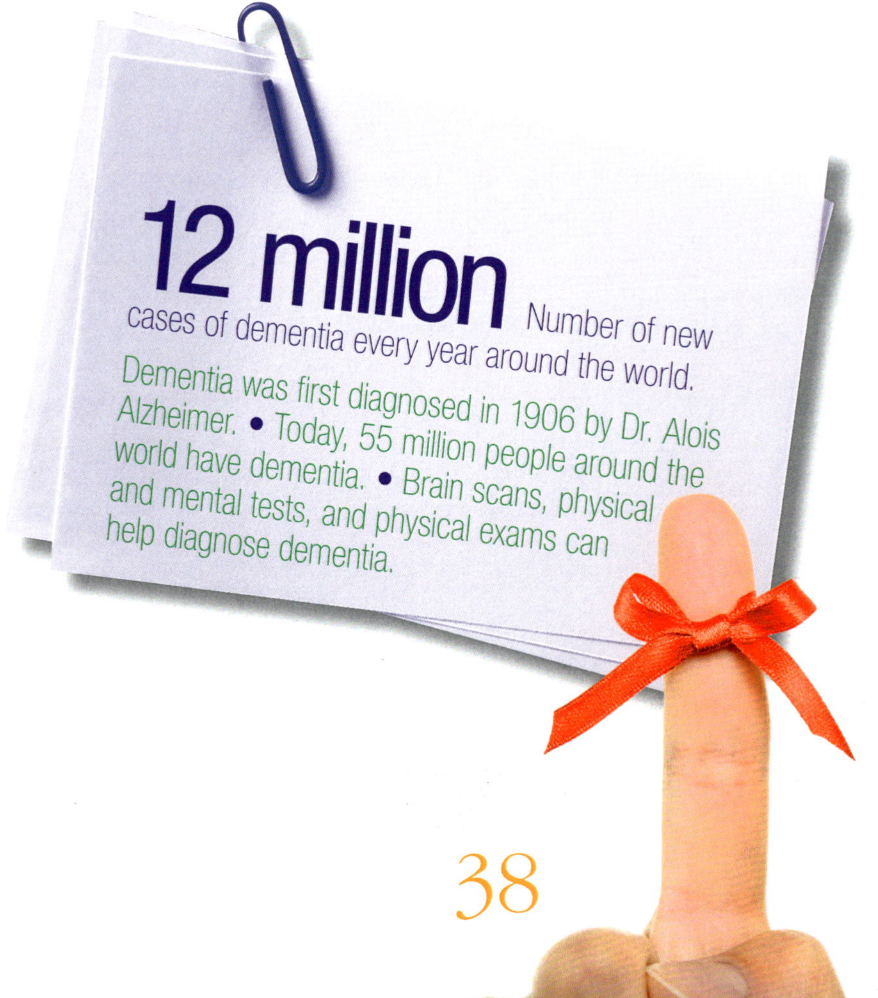

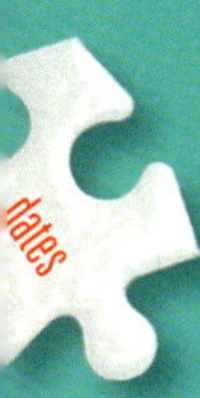

People with Alzheimer's often forget basic facts and memories about their life.

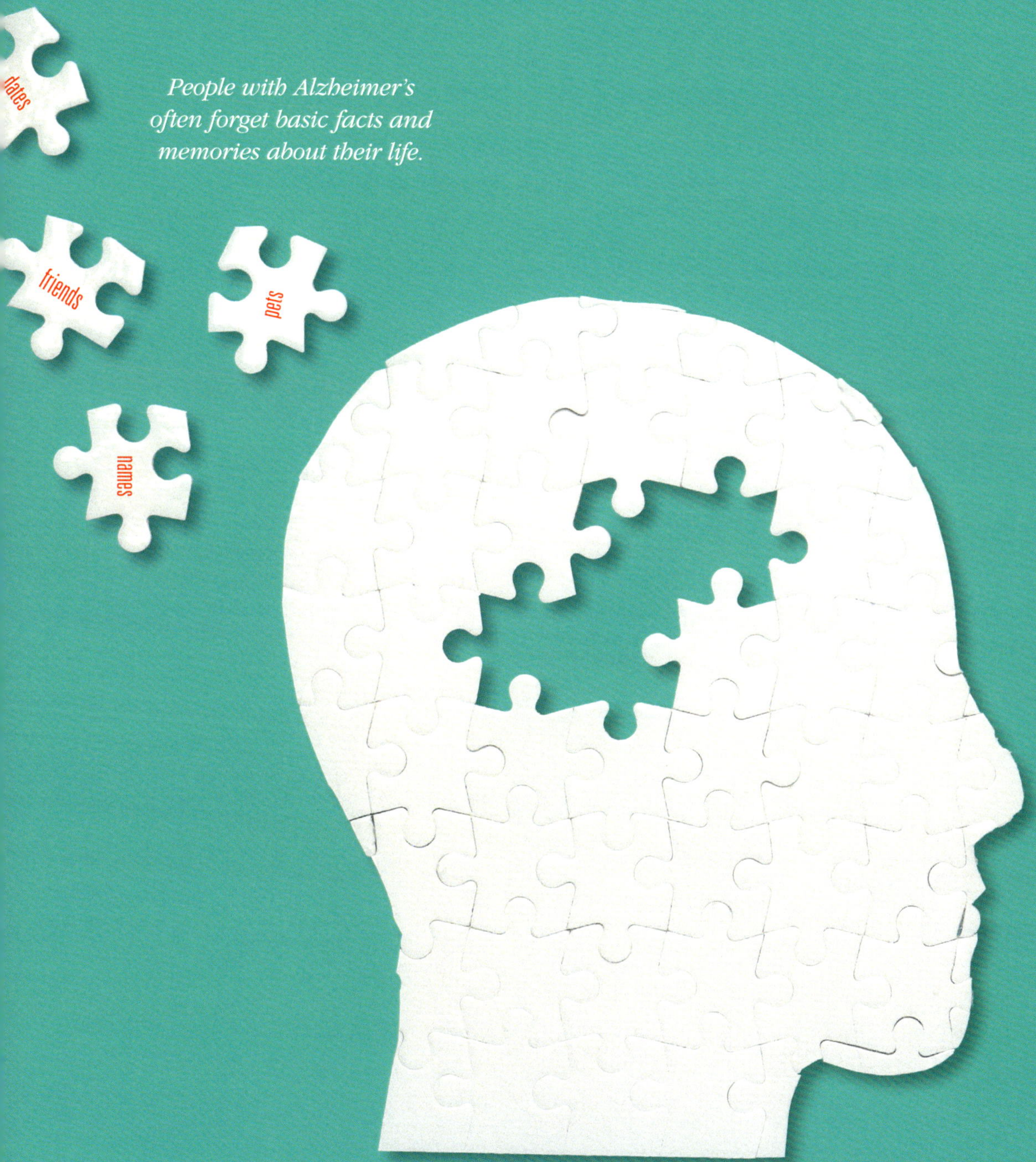

AI Robots Make Hospital *Work Easier*

12

Hospitals are huge places. Many US hospitals have more than 250 beds. They average almost 354,000 square feet (32,900 square meters.) That's a lot of space! Beds need to be changed. Meals and medicine need to be delivered. Waste needs to be removed.

Aetheon's TUG robots can cover that distance with ease. They have a user-friendly **interface**. Even people with no training can use TUG. The bots can follow a schedule. They can also be called to a spot with an app.

TUGs can carry large loads. One model can hold up to 1,000 pounds (453 kilograms). This saves a person time making trips back and forth. The robots can handle delicate laboratory samples. They can safely get rid of dangerous material. One big plus is that they can travel into **contagious** areas. This lowers the risk of spreading germs.

TUGs have various sensors and AI programming. They can plan routes. They can react to real-time situations. This shaves minutes off deliveries. Future bots may be able to make decisions. They will sort orders and deliver the important ones first. They may even communicate directly with patients.

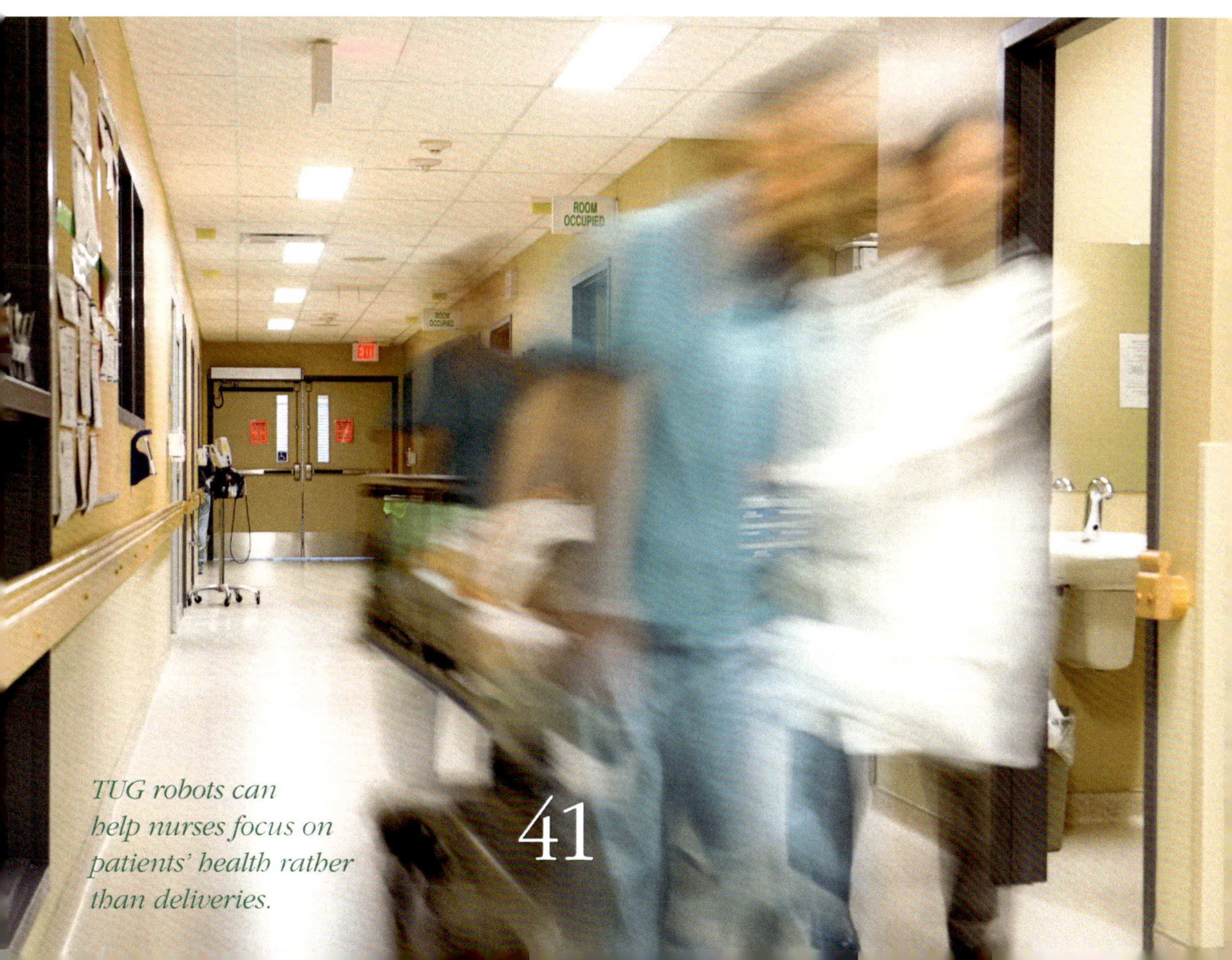

TUG robots can help nurses focus on patients' health rather than deliveries.

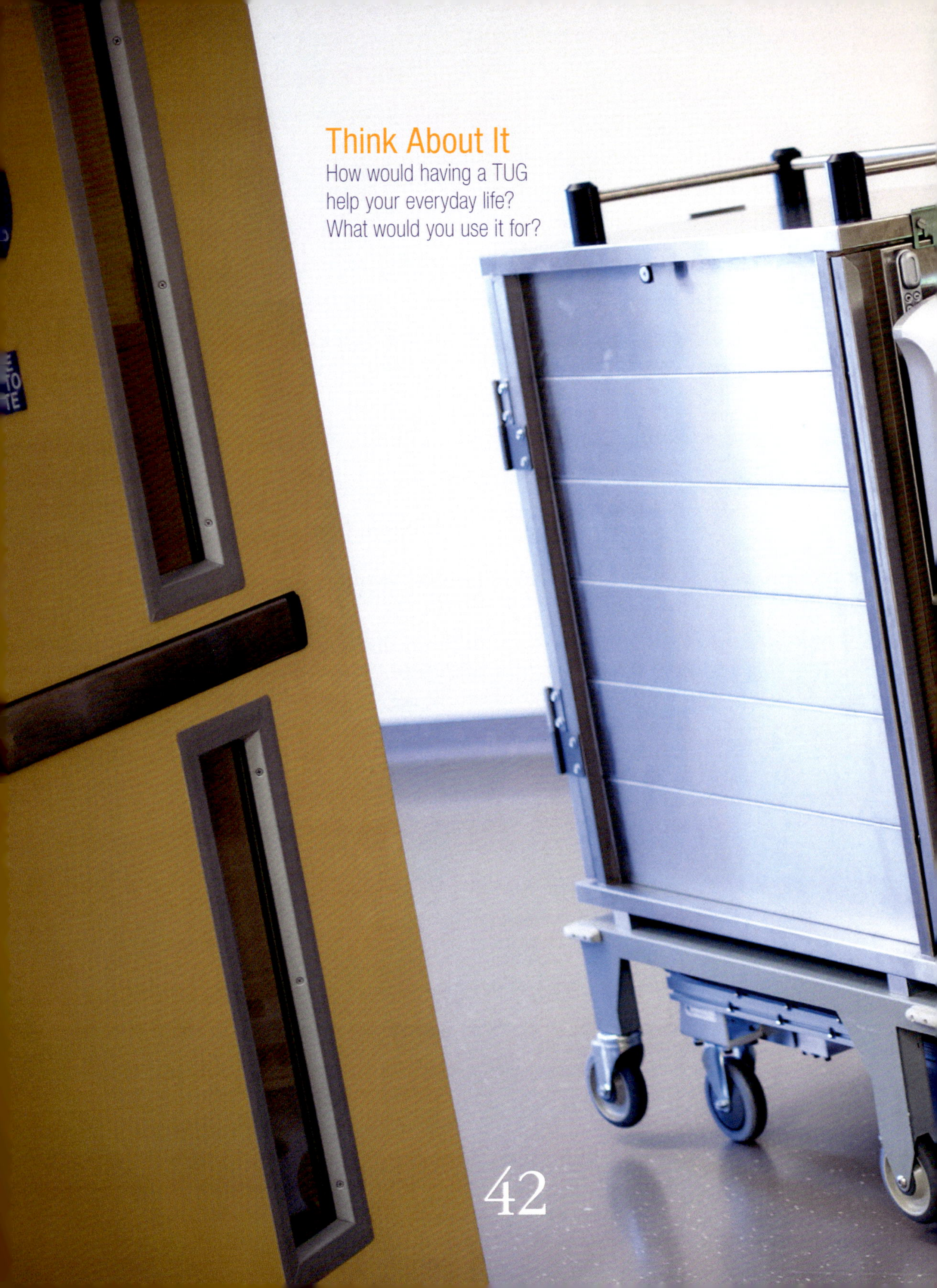

Think About It

How would having a TUG help your everyday life? What would you use it for?

DINEX CARLISLE
TUG
4 Number of miles (6.4 km) an average hospital worker walks every shift.
Some walk more than double this distance. • TUG can work for 10 hours on a single charge. • The first TUG was put to work in 2004.

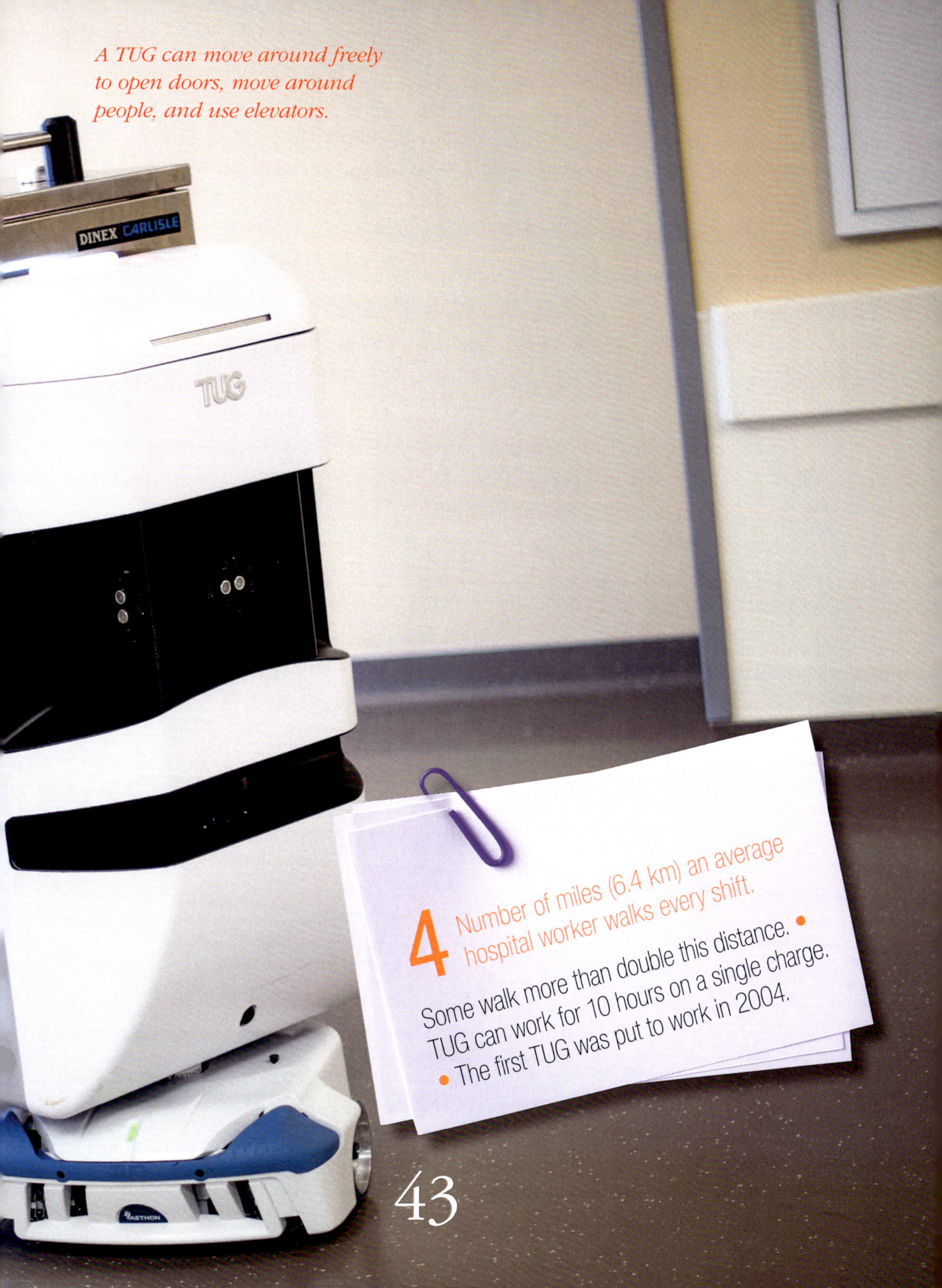

A TUG can move around freely to open doors, move around people, and use elevators.

Fact

- It can take 10 years to develop a new drug. It is also very expensive. The biotech company Exscientia is using AI to speed up the process. Usually, drugs are tested on patients. They must be tested one at a time. Exscentia is much faster and safer. Their AI is also designing new drugs. It predicts the effects of those drugs on people. It throws out any that look unsafe.

- Pet medicine is using AI too. Owners can use ChatGPT to diagnose their pets. Then they know if it's a big or small problem. There's also an AI app called VetGPT. It gives even more detailed vet responses.

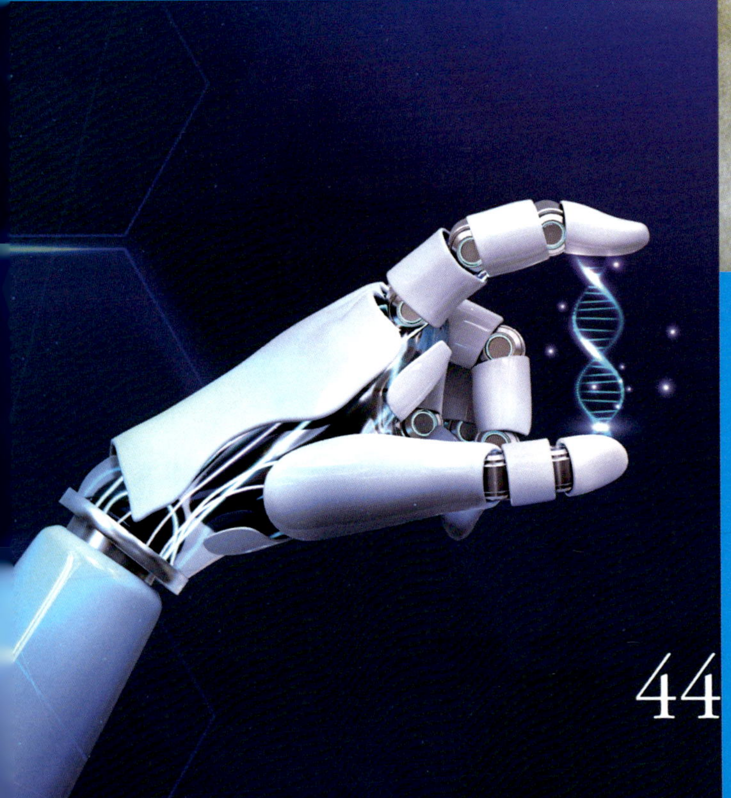

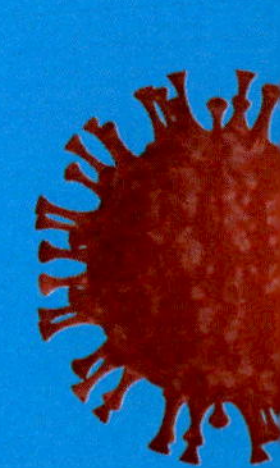

Sheet

• AI is even used to treat everyday illnesses. It has been used to track the effectiveness of over-the-counter flu medication. It can predict whether you have COVID-19 or the flu.

• Around 380 viruses live in and on your body right now. In 2025, the Human Virome Project took samples from thousands of volunteers. They ran them past AI. They hope to learn about viruses that live in our bodies.

• People without a limb may have trouble adjusting to a prosthetic. AI pairs with haptic sensors to connect signals from a person's brain to their limb. The more the limb is worn, the more AI can figure out how to optimize its features.

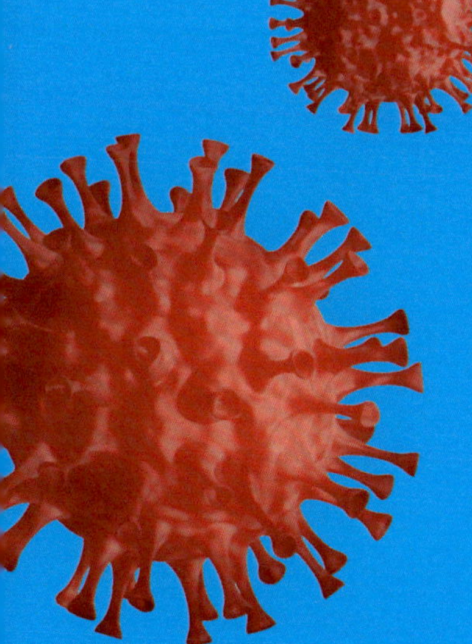

Glossary

bias
A tendency to believe that some people or ideas are better than others that usually results in treating some people unfairly.

biometric
Body measurements and calculations related to human characteristics and features.

contagious
Relating to an illness that can spread from one being to another.

critical
Relating to or involving a great danger of death.

diagnose
To recognize a disease, illness, or injury by signs and symptoms.

implant
Something placed in a person's body by means of surgery.

insurance
The business of providing an amount of money to a person who makes regular payments as part of an agreement to cover medical costs.

interface
A system that controls the way information is shown and how the user is able to work with the computer.

pharmacist
A person who prepares and sell drugs and medicines that a doctor has prescribed.

predict
To say something will happen in the future.

rural
Relating to the countryside and the people who live there.

specialist
A doctor who deals with health problems that relate to a specific area of medicine.

telemedicine
A virtual doctor's visit using a device with video call.

tissue
A mass of cells enclosed with another substance that forms the basic structural materials of plants and animals.

transcribe
To write down something that is spoken.

vital sign
A measurement such as heart rate, blood pressure, and temperature that can be tracked to help determine a person's health.

For More Information

Books

Harris, Beatrice. *Jobs in Artificial Intelligence.* New York: Cavendish Square Publishing, 2024.

Loughrey, Anita. *Body & Health Tech.* Minneapolis: Bearport Publishing Company, 2025.

Ventura, Marne. *12 Questions about Artificial Intelligence.* Mankato, MN: Black Rabbit Books, 2026.

Websites

Humans and AI Working Together
tpt.pbslearningmedia.org/resource/humans-and-ai-working-together-video/crash-course-artificial-intelligence/

Robot that Watched Surgery Videos Performs with Skills of Human Doctor
hub.jhu.edu/2024/11/11/surgery-robots-trained-with-videos/

About the Author

Mari Bolte is a writer and editor who enjoys wondering about where the future of technology will take us. Whether it's exploring outer space or thinking about how AI can make her life easier, one might say she has her head in "the cloud."

Index

TOP RANK is published by Black Rabbit Books, P.O. Box 227, Mankato, MN, 56002.

• Designed by Danny Nanos • Photographs © Dreamstime/Ai8075, cover, 1; Freepik/Bogac Dalkiran, 45; Getty Images/Just_Super, 26, Noah Berger/Bloomberg, 40, 42–43; Shutterstock/Agenturfotografin, 4, Aleksandar Malivuk, 34-35, Alex Photo Stock, 8, Andrei Shumskiy, 37, 38, April stock, 13, 21, AtlasStudio, 39, AXL, 36, Belinda Pretorius, 48, Dmitry Naumov, 31, doomu, 11, Gorodenkoff, 2–3, 17, 20, Have a nice day Photo, 5, janews, 29, Javier Brosch, 44, Jolygon, 46–47, Kateryna Kon, 10, Koliadzynska Iryna, 10, Komsan Loonprom, 8–9, Ljupco Smokovski, 16, Martin Bergsma, 31, Matteo Migliorati, 44–45, Maxxionn, 14, metamorworks, 14, Motionblur Studios, 2, 18–19, Mr Doomits, 27, nimito, 32–33, Phonlamai Photo, 22–23, Prostock-studio, 28, Puwadol Jaturawutthichai, 36, Rawpixel.com, 44, Skrypnykov Dmytro, 25, Summit Art Creations, 7, 11, Tyler Olson, 41, vectorfusionart, 15, Who is Danny, 12, Zdenka Darula, 6, 501room, 27 • Printed in the United States of America. **Library of Congress Cataloging-in-Publication Data:** Names: Bolte, Mari author | Title: 12 uses for artificial intelligence in healthcare / Mari Bolte. | Other titles: Twelve uses for artificial intelligence in healthcare | Description: Mankato, MN: Top Rank is an imprint of Black Rabbit Books, [2026] | Series: AI in the world | Includes bibliographical references and index. | Audience: Ages 9–13 | Audience: Grades 4–6 | Identifiers: LCCN 2025021454 (print) | LCCN 2025021455 (ebook) | ISBN 9781645825166 library binding | ISBN 9781645825340 paperback | ISBN 9781645825524 ebook | Subjects: LCSH: Artificial intelligence—Medical applications—Juvenile literature | Classification: LCC R859.7.A78 B65 2026 (print) | LCC R859.7.A78 (ebook) | LC record available at https://lccn.loc.gov/2025021454 | LC ebook record available at https://lccn.loc.gov/202502145